Hand Burns

Guest Editor

MATTHEW B. KLEIN, MD, MS, FACS

HAND CLINICS

www.hand.theclinics.com

November 2009 • Volume 25 • Number 4

SAUNDERS an imprint of ELSEVIER, Inc.

W.B. SAUNDERS COMPANY
A Division of Elsevier Inc.

1600 John F. Kennedy Blvd. • Suite 1800 • Philadelphia, Pennsylvania 19103

http://www.theclinics.com

HAND CLINICS Volume 25, Number 4
November 2009 ISSN 0749-0712, ISBN-13: 978-1-4377-1224-7, ISBN-10: 1-4377-1224-X

Editor: Debora Dellapena
Developmental Editor: Theresa Collier

Hand Clinics (ISSN 0749-0712) is published quarterly by Elsevier Inc., 360 Park Avenue South, New York, NY 10010-1710. Months of publication are February, May, August, and November. Application to mail at periodicals postage rates is pending at New York, NY and at additional mailing offices. Subscription price is $282.00 per year (domestic individuals), $446.00 per year (domestic institutions), $144.00 per year (domestic students/residents), $321.00 per year (Canadian individuals), $510.00 per year (Canadian institutions), $383.00 per year (international individuals), $510.00 per year (international institutions), and $189.00 per year (international and Canadian students/residents). Foreign air speed delivery is included in all *Clinics* subscription prices. All prices are subject to change without notice. **POSTMASTER:** Send address changes to *Hand Clinics*, Elsevier Health Sciences Division, Subscription Customer Service, 3251 Riverport Lane, Maryland Heights, MO 63043. Customer Service (orders, claims, online, change of address): Elsevier Health Sciences Division, Subscription Customer Service, 3251 Riverport Lane, Maryland Heights, MO 63043. Tel: 1-800-654-2452 (U.S. and Canada); 314-447-8871 (outside U.S. and Canada). Fax: 314-447-8029. E-mail: journalscustomerservice-usa@elsevier.com (for print support); journalsonlinesupport-usa@elsevier.com (for online support).

Reprints. For copies of 100 or more of articles in this publication, please contact the Commercial Reprints Department, Elsevier Inc., 360 Park Avenue South, New York, New York 10010-1710. Tel.: 212-633-3812; Fax: 212-462-1935; E-mail: reprints@elsevier.com.

Hand Clinics is covered in *MEDLINE/PubMed (Index Medicus), Current Contents/Clinical Medicine, EMBASE/Excerpta Medica,* and *ISI/BIOMED.*

Printed and bound by CPI Group (UK) Ltd, Croydon, CR0 4YY

Transferred to Digital Print 2011

Contributors

GUEST EDITOR

MATTHEW B. KLEIN, MD, MS, FACS
David and Nancy Auth-Washington Research
Foundation Endowed Chair for Restorative
Burn Surgery; and Associate Director; and
Associate Professor, University of Washington
Regional Burn Center, Division of Plastic
Surgery, Department of Surgery, Harborview
Medical Center, Seattle, Washington

AUTHORS

DAVID H. AHRENHOLZ, MD
The Burn Center, Department of Trauma and
General Surgery, Regions Hospital; Associate
Professor, Department of Surgery, University
of Minnesota, St. Paul, Minnesota

BRETT D. ARNOLDO, MD
Associate Professor, Department of Surgery,
University of Texas Southwestern Medical
Center, Dallas, Texas

RUDOLF F. BUNTIC, MD
Clinical Assistant Professor (Affiliated),
Department of Surgery, Stanford University
School of Medicine, Stanford, California;
The Buncke Clinic, Davies Medical Center,
San Francisco, California

WILLIAM S. DEWEY, PT, CHT, OCS
Clinical Coordinator, Army Burn Center, Burn
Rehabilitation, United States Army Institute of
Surgical Research, Fort Sam Houston, Texas

JIE DING, PhD
Research Associate, Division of Plastic
and Reconstructive Surgery, Department
of Surgery, University of Alberta, Edmonton,
Canada

NICOLE S. GIBRAN, MD
Professor and Director, University of
Washington Regional Burn Center, Department
of Surgery, Harborview Medical Center,
Seattle, Washington

WILLIAM L. HICKERSON, MD
Professor of Plastic Surgery, Department
of Plastic Surgery, University of Tennessee
Health Science Center; Director, Firefighters'
Regional Burn Center, Memphis, Tennessee

KEIJIRO HORI, MD
Post Doctoral Fellow, Division of Plastic and
Reconstructive Surgery, Department of
Surgery, University of Alberta, Edmonton,
Canada

KAMRUN JENABZADEH, MD
Surgery Resident, University of Minnesota,
St. Paul, Minnesota

YVONNE L. KARANAS, MD
Director, Burn Center; Associate Chief
of Plastic Surgery, Santa Clara Valley Medical
Center, San Jose, California; Clinical Assistant
Professor, Department of Surgery, Stanford
University School of Medicine, Stanford,
California

MATTHEW B. KLEIN, MD, MS, FACS
David and Nancy Auth-Washington Research
Foundation Endowed Chair for Restorative
Burn Surgery; and Associate Director; and
Associate Professor, University of Washington
Regional Burn Center, Division of Plastic
Surgery, Department of Surgery, Harborview
Medical Center, Seattle, Washington

KAREN KOWALSKE, MD
Professor and Chair, Department of Physical Medicine and Rehabilitation, University of Texas Southwestern Medical Center, Dallas, Texas

PETER KWAN, MD
Graduate Student, Division of Plastic and Reconstructive Surgery, Department of Surgery, University of Alberta, Edmonton, Canada

RICHARD BENJAMIN LOU, MD
Burn Fellow, Firefighters' Regional Burn Center, University of Tennessee Health Science Center, Memphis, Tennessee

ROBERT L. McCAULEY, MD
Professor, Surgery and Pediatrics, University of Texas Medical Branch; Chief of Plastic and Reconstructive Surgery, Shriners Hospitals for Children, Galveston, Texas

WM J. MOHR, MD
The Burn Center, Department of Trauma and General Surgery, Regions Hospital; Assistant Professor, Department of Surgery, University of Minnesota, St. Paul, Minnesota

MERILYN L. MOORE, PT
Manager, Rehabilitation Therapies and Burn Plastics Clinic, University of Washington Burn Center, Harborview Medical Center, Seattle, Washington

TINA L. PALMIERI, MD, FACS, FCCM
Shriners Hospital for Children Northern California, University of California Davis, Sacramento, California

GARY F. PURDUE, MD
Professor, Department of Surgery, University of Texas Southwestern Medical Center, Dallas, Texas

REGINALD L. RICHARD, MS, PT
Clinical Research Coordinator, Army Burn Center, Burn Rehabilitation, United States Army Institute of Surgical Research, Fort Sam Houston, Texas

JOSE STERLING, MD
Fellow, University of Washington Regional Burn Center, Harborview Medical Center, Seattle, Washington

EDWARD E. TREDGET, MD, MSc, FRCSC
Professor, Division of Plastic and Reconstructive Surgery, Department of Surgery; Division of Critical Care, Department of Surgery, University of Alberta, Edmonton, Canada

Contents

Karen Kowalske

> Overall outcome following hand burns is closely related to the depth of injury. Although even full-thickness burns tend to result in favorable outcomes, injuries to the deeper structures may result in some degree of impairment. Reviewing the existing literature on hand burns clearly demonstrates the need for validated measurement tools for the evaluation of hand burn outcomes.

Hand Clinics

THE CLINICS ARE NOW AVAILABLE ONLINE!

Access your subscription at:
www.theclinics.com

Preface

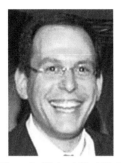

Matthew B. Klein, MD, MS, FACS
Guest Editor

Advances in critical care and resuscitation have significantly improved survival following thermal injury. In 2009 survival following extensive burn injury has become the rule rather than the exception. Given this increase in survival, there has been an evolution in the emphasis in clinical care of the burn patient toward optimizing the function and appearance of those that survive their injuries. The hand plays a critical role in an individual's interactions with his or her environment. Hand function is critical to completing activities of daily living and the conduct of vocational and leisure activities.

Thermal injuries of the hand can vary from superficial wounds that readily heal without long-term consequence to deep injuries that threaten the viability of the hand. Management of hand burns requires a multidisciplinary team of physicians, nurses, therapists, vocational counselors, and occasionally rehabilitation psychologists. This issue of *Hand Clinics* is dedicated to the management of burn injuries of the hand, from the straightforward to the complex, and provides detailed information on management of each. Authors of each article have spent a significant portion of their careers working with burn patients and the content of the articles reflects the experience of a working life dedicated to the optimal outcome of those who sustain burn injuries.

Matthew B. Klein, MD, MS, FACS
University of Washington Regional Burn Center
Division of Plastic Surgery
Department of Surgery
Harborview Medical Center
325 9th Avenue
Box 359796, Seattle, WA 98104, USA

E-mail address:
mbklein@u.washington.edu (M.B. Klein)

Hand Clin 25 (2009) ix
doi:10.1016/j.hcl.2009.08.001

hand.theclinics.com

Acute Management of Hand Burns

Jose Sterling, MD[a], Nicole S. Gibran, MD[b],*,
Matthew B. Klein, MD, MS, FACS[c]

KEYWORDS

- Hand burns • Acute • Wound management
- Chemical injuries • Excision and grafting

Hand burns are common, either isolated or associated with other thermal injuries. Even though the relative body surface area of the hand is small, burns can significantly affect functional capacity and quality of life.[1–3] Classically, the focus of care for patients with major burns evolved around grafting of larger body areas, and little priority was given to the acute management or rehabilitation of burned hands.[4] However, during the past 30 years, techniques of early excision and grafting have significantly improved survival after burn injury[5] and, accordingly, shifted emphasis toward optimizing functional outcomes of the burn survivor. Therefore, preservation of hand function has received increased attention. Currently, standard burn care includes an aggressive, multidisciplinary approach to the hand, with care coordinated among experienced physical and occupational therapists as well as burn surgeons and plastic surgeons, at specialized burn centers. For these reasons, the American Burn Association has included hand burns in its Burn Center Referral Criteria (www.ameriburn.org; **Box 1**).[6]

INITIAL EXAMINATION AND HISTORY

A detailed discussion and analysis of the systemic effects of burn injuries are beyond the scope of this article. Initial evaluation and fluid resuscitation should follow the guidelines given in the American Burn Association's Advanced Burn Life Support (ABLS) manual.[7] Management of patient critical illness and response to injury always takes precedence over the hand burn. However, even during the resuscitation phase of care, early attention to face, ear, and hand injuries can be crucial to successful eventual outcomes. Patient and injury history should include the mechanism and circumstances surrounding the injury. If possible, this history should include patient occupation, hand dominance, and history of preexisting extremity injury.

Physical examination of the burned hand should focus on determining the extent of injury and vascular supply. High-risk injuries such as circumferential burns, crush injuries, and lacerations can easily lead to vascular compromise. On examination, warning signs of vascular insufficiency are diminished pulses, lack of or sluggish capillary refill, and skin that is cool to palpation.[4] The importance of checking for adequate vascular perfusion to the hand cannot be overemphasized, but it can be extremely difficult in the burned hand, given discoloration and damage to normal anatomy. Typically, compromised perfusion is not an issue with superficial and partial-thickness hand burns. However, full-thickness eschar can compromise hand and digit perfusion. Edema secondary to major burn injury and the subsequent fluid resuscitation also compromise perfusion to the hand and digits. Therefore, extremity elevation and close neurovascular monitoring is necessary.

[a] University of Washington Regional Burn Center, Harborview Medical Center, Box 359796, 325 Ninth Avenue, Seattle, WA 98104, USA
[b] University of Washington Regional Burn Center, Department of Surgery, Harborview Medical Center, Box 359796, 325 Ninth Avenue, Seattle, WA 98104, USA
[c] University of Washington Regional Burn Center, Division of Plastic Surgery, Department of Surgery, Harborview Medical Center, Box 359796, 325 Ninth Avenue, Seattle, WA 98104, USA
* Corresponding author.
E-mail address: nicoleg@u.washington.edu (N.S. Gibran).

Hand Clin 25 (2009) 453–459
doi:10.1016/j.hcl.2009.06.010
0749-0712/09/$ – see front matter © 2009 Elsevier Inc. All rights reserved.

Box 1
American Burn Association transfer criteria

1. Second degree burns (partial thickness) of greater than 10% of the body surface area
2. Third degree burns (full thickness) in any age group
3. Inhalation injury
4. Burns involving the face, hands, feet, genitalia, major joints, or perineum
5. Electrical injury or burn (including lightning)
6. Burns associated with trauma or complicating medical conditions
7. Chemical burns
8. Burn injury in patients with preexisting medical disorders that could complicate management, prolong recovery, or affect mortality
9. Patients in hospitals without qualified personnel or equipment for the care of children
10. Burn injury in patients who will require special social, emotional, or rehabilitative intervention

Modified from American Burn Association Burn Center referral criteria (http://www.ameriburn.org/BurnCenterReferralCriteria.pdf); with permission.

The hand should be warm and should have a normal capillary refill time of 2 to 3 seconds. A hand with inadequate perfusion will be cold, may lack pulses, and will exhibit sensory and motor neuropathy, often leading to a clawed position on examination.[8] However, hand temperature may be misleading in a hypothermic patient. Hand and digit perfusion can be confirmed by the presence of a Doppler signal over the ulnar and radial arteries and the palmar arch and digital arteries.[4,9] Any evidence of hypoperfusion in conjunction with a hand or forearm burn should lead to consideration and timely performance of escharotomies to prevent ischemic necrosis of the hand.[8–10]

ESCHAROTOMY

The purpose of escharotomy is to improve perfusion by releasing the pressure created by the restrictive burned tissue. Escharotomies to the forearm and hand can be performed with electrocautery or a scalpel. This procedure is typically performed at the bedside under sterile conditions. The endpoint of escharotomy is release of the eschar, expansion of the underlying tissue compartments, and subsequent return of perfusion. Escharotomy incisions can be visible, and they make subsequent burn excision more challenging or aesthetically unacceptable if the burn heals without surgery. It is important that the escharotomy incision extends only through eschar, and not into the fat or fascia. Forearm escharotomies involve axial incisions at the radial and ulnar aspect extending to the metacarpophalangeal joints of the first and fifth digits (**Fig. 1**);[11,12] these incisions should be performed with the extremity in the anatomic position. Hand escharotomies are performed with incisions through the eschar from the base of the hand to the metacarpal heads in the intermetacarpal spaces (**Fig. 2**) to avoid unnecessary exposure of tendon. The use of digital escharotomies is highly debated.[13] However, the risk of exposing or injuring digital nerves, vessels, and tendons likely outweighs any potential benefits. There is insufficient muscle to prevent significant rhabdomyolysis, and burns of the digits are likely sufficiently deep that the burn itself has injured the underlying structures.

Electrical injuries may require fasciotomies. In these cases, fasciotomies are performed using volar and dorsal incisions over the forearm.[14,15] The potential benefit of simultaneous prophylactic carpal tunnel release at the time of fasciotomies after electrical injury is debatable.[16] Full details of electrical injury management can be found elsewhere in this issue.

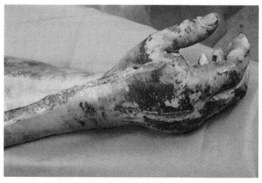

Fig. 1. Forearm escharotomy extending to the hand.

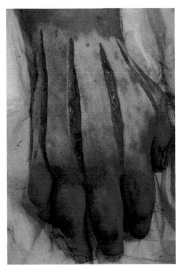

Fig. 2. Hand escharotomies placed in the intermetacarpal spaces.

WOUND MANAGEMENT

At the time of initial evaluation, it is important to debride any loose or thin blisters and remove any foreign material from the wounds before applying dressings. If intact blisters do not limit hand range of motion or functional activity, they can be left intact; they make excellent wound coverage. The wide variety of dressing materials available today for burn care is not addressed here.[17]

The goals of all dressings are to prevent infection, to prevent water and heat loss, and to promote epithelialization; they should also be easy to apply and relatively painless and inexpensive. For deep partial-thickness and full-thickness burns, application of silver sulfadiazine followed by a dry gauze dressing is soothing and simple. For shallow partial-thickness burns and for burns in which epithelialization has begun, a regimen of nonadherent greasy gauze combined with bacitracin is useful and simple. However, the paramount principle in dressing a hand burn is to facilitate motion. Therefore, any dressing must allow the patient to fully use and exercise the hand.

The hand burn should be continually reevaluated for healing progress. During the 'wait and watch' period or if nonoperative treatment is pursued, aggressive exercise and hand therapy should be initiated soon after injury and continued daily to minimize edema and maximize range of motion. If the patient is intubated or is otherwise unable to actively range the hand and digits, then passive range of motion should occur. Hand burns that are not likely to heal within 21 days of injury should be managed by excision and skin grafting

as time and patient stability permit. Prompt excision and subsequent grafting of burn wounds has resulted in less hypertrophic scarring, debilitating contractures, and need for reconstruction with overall improved patient outcome.[4,8,9,18] Often in patients with major burns, the timing for definitive excision and grafting may be deferred by the need to excise other injuries. However, for this subset of patients, early excision with placement of a skin substitute while waiting for donor site availability is beneficial.[19–22]

Palm contact burns warrant special attention. Palm contact burns typically occur in young children and result in deep partial-thickness palm burns. Despite many advocates in the literature for the idea that such burns should be excised and grafted immediately with thick skin grafts, the concern for maintaining the irreplaceable cutaneous-fascial attachments and the pacinian corpuscles that make grip and tactile senses specialized has led to the approach to manage palm burns nonoperatively.[23] However, this approach requires emphasis on an aggressive exercise plan and possible extension splinting to maintain range of motion and to prevent contraction during the healing process.[3,23] If the wound shows evidence of granulation tissue formation rather than epithelialization or if the hand begins to contract at all, excision and grafting should be scheduled. This care plan should be initiated immediately and must always engage parents for continuing therapy at home.

EXCISION AND GRAFTING OF HAND BURNS

Tourniquets should be used to minimize blood loss during excision. Tangential excision is performed to viable subcutaneous tissue. For areas that are difficult to excise, such as web spaces or cuticles, the Versajet (Smith & Nephew, London, United Kingdom) water dissector can be used to perform the tangential excision.[24] Given the relatively thin skin and subcutaneous tissue layer on the dorsum of the hand, every effort must be made to ensure that underlying tendons or joints are not exposed.

Once excision is complete, tissue viability should be verified after deflation of the tourniquet by demonstrating a diffusely bleeding bed. Epinephrine-soaked Telfa dressings (Kendall Company, Mansfield, Massachusetts) and epinephrine-soaked lap pads (concentration 1:10,000) are applied to the wound bed for 10 minutes to achieve hemostasis with a pressure dressing. Electrocautery for punctate bleeding and fibrin sealant facilitate hemostasis.

To optimize function, durability, and aesthetics, sheet grafts should always be used for hands and wrists unless there is such a paucity of donor sites that this plan compromises lifesaving coverage of other major burn wounds. The anterolateral thigh is a preferred donor site in adult patients and older children because of ease of intraoperative access, postoperative care, and ability to hide it under a pair of shorts or a skirt. In younger children, the authors attempt to use the buttocks, with care taken to ensure that harvest occurs in the area within the confines of a diaper. Skin is harvested using a dermatome—either air or electric. In cases where the entire hand requires grafting, a dermatome with a 6-in guard can minimize the number of graft junctions. Split-thickness sheet grafts should be harvested slightly thicker than grafts for other sites to ensure durability and elasticity (0.012 in for dorsal hands and 0.015–0.018 in for palms). A study evaluating thicker grafts for dorsal hand burns demonstrated no benefit in function or patient satisfaction when compared with full-thickness grafts.[25] In small burns, especially palm burns or web spaces, where full-thickness grafts are beneficial, the inguinal crease or flank provides adequate skin and can be closed primarily.

Grafts can be affixed to the wound in several ways. One ideal approach is to tack the grafts with two or three absorbable sutures at graft junctures or corners and to apply aerosolized fibrin glue to the wound bed;[26] the fibrin sealant promotes graft adherence and minimizes postoperative collections of wound exudate or blood. The graft adhesion can be reinforced with small strips of Hypafix tape (Smith & Nephew, London, United Kingdom) (**Fig. 3**).[27] A thin layer of a nonadherent material should be placed over the graft itself, followed by a conforming wrap and resting splint application. Grafting should always be performed with the hand in that same position as it will be during postoperative immobilization (5–7 days). Careful attention should be paid to ensure that the thumb-index web space is as wide as possible to minimize contracture, which commonly occurs at this site. Grafting the fingers in slight flexion maximizes the length of graft placed on the wounds and facilitates postoperative exercising.

Dressings are briefly removed on postoperative day 1 to examine the graft for underlying seromas or hematomas (**Fig. 4**). Small nicks in the graft using a #11 blade evacuate fluid collections. If collections are minimal, dressings are reapplied until postoperative day 5, when the graft is assessed for adequacy of adherence and graft take. A lighter dressing can be applied at this time over a layer of greasy gauze to prevent adherence of dressings to the still-fragile sheet graft; if postoperative swelling persists, the graft can be wrapped with an elastic dressing such as Coban (3M, St Paul, Minnesota). Passive and active range of motion should be initiated at this time.

A silver-impregnated dressing is an easy postoperative dressing plan for the donor site. Covered firmly for 24 hours postoperatively, it can then be exposed to the air to dry. The dry edges lift as the wound bed epithelializes and can be trimmed circumferentially until donor site healing is complete. For buttocks donor sites in infants and toddlers, silver sulfadiazine can be applied directly into the diaper without a dressing and reapplied with soiling.

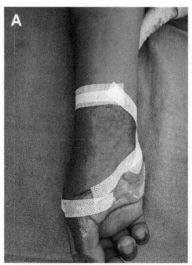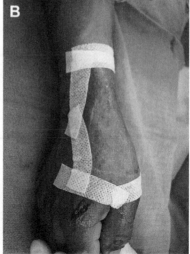

Fig. 3. Hypafix tape fixation of a skin graft to the hand and forearm (*A*) and (*B*).

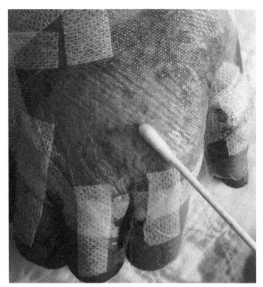

Fig. 4. Skin graft evaluation on postoperative day one. Any fluid collections are drained to prevent graft loss.

DEEP HAND BURNS

Given the relatively thin soft tissue coverage overlying the hand, deep flame or contact thermal injuries can result in exposed tendons, bones, joints, and neurovascular structures. Typically, simple skin graft coverage alone is not feasible, and flap coverage may be required. Because patients with extensor tendon loss will ultimately develop severe flexion contractures, early arthrodesis using Kirschner wires at the time of soft tissue coverage may be necessary. This prevents the subsequent, inevitable contractures, and allows the patient to enter the rehabilitation phase of their injury with a stable and functionally positioned hand. Options for soft tissue coverage depends on the location and depth of other injuries. Local tissue coverage for the hand and digits can include the radial forearm fascia or fasciocutaneous flap; however, the forearm fascia is rarely spared in deep burns of the hand. A standard Allen test is needed before raising the flap, to ensure patency of the ulnar and radial artery to the hand. In addition, Doppler verification of the presence of an intact superficial palmar arch is important. Alternatively, pedicled flaps from the chest, abdomen, flank, or groin can be used if available. The hand and/or digits can be placed under a flap raised at the subfascial level and left in place for 2 to 3 weeks. At the time of flap division, the hand can be released with either transfer of the entire flap as hand coverage and grafting of the abdominal defect or division of the flap just superficial to the fascia and skin grafting to the hand and suturing

of the chest or abdominal skin and subcutaneous tissue back into place. A final soft-tissue coverage option would be a microvascular tissue transfer, which is especially useful if the deep burn injury extends to the forearm and eliminates the option of local tissue flap. An ideal flap provides thin, contoured, pliable, and durable coverage for hand injuries. Options include the contralateral radial forearm fascia, the dorsalis pedis fascia or temporoparietal fascia; perforator flaps, such as the thin anterolateral thigh perforator flap, have also been described for hand coverage after burn injury.

AMPUTATION

In the case of severe hand burns, salvage of the hand and/or digits may not be feasible or practical. Discussions with the patient regarding realistic and functional results of reconstruction are essential. Careful assessment of the extent of tendon, joint, and bone damage, weighing options for soft-tissue coverage with either skin grafts or tissue flaps, must be discussed. The ultimate goal of optimal hand function should guide decisions of digit or hand preservation.

Digit or hand amputations are rarely emergent, particularly if there is any chance of deep tissue viability or the potential for adequate coverage with a local or distant flap. A delayed amputation can always be performed if the graft or flap fails. Furthermore, critically ill patients may benefit from inclusion in decision-making regarding amputations; therefore waiting until they can participate in the discussion may be ideal. Once the level of digit or limb viability has been declared, acute amputation at a level of normal tissue is indicated. Whereas length should be preserved to the greatest extent possible, functional outcome should be the priority. For example an insensate, immobile digit is less functional in many cases than an amputation.

CHEMICAL BURNS

Chemical burns have been traditionally classified as either acid burns or alkali (base) burns. The severity of chemical injuries typically depends on the composition of the agent, concentration of the agent, and contact duration with the agent. Alkali burns typically cause more severe injury than acid burns because alkaline agents cause a liquefaction necrosis that allows the alkali to penetrate deeper, extending the area of injury. Chemical injuries most commonly involve the hand.

The first step in managing a chemical injury is removal of the inciting agent. Clothes and shoes that have been contaminated should be carefully removed. Skin areas in contact with the chemical agent should be irrigated copiously with water. Adequate irrigation can be verified by checking the skin pH. It is critical that neutralization of the inciting agent should never be attempted because this will produce an exothermic reaction that will superimpose a thermal injury on top of the chemical injury. Burns resulting from chemical powders are the one exception to the rule of water irrigation because the water can activate the chemical. The powder should first be dusted off, and then irrigation can occur. Occasionally, the burned individual may not know specifically with which agent they were working, and therefore it may be necessary to contact a plant manager or the manufacturer of the suspected inciting agent.

Certain chemical agents have specific treatments. For example, hydrofluoric acid (HF) requires specific mention. HF is commonly used in the glass and silicon chip industries and in several industrial cleaning solutions. HF readily penetrates the skin and continues to injure tissue until it comes in contact with a calcium source, likely bone. Given the ability of the fluoride ion to chelate calcium, patients with even small HF burns are at risk for the development of hypocalcemia that can be severe enough to have deleterious cardiac effects. The use of calcium is the most effective treatment agent. Calcium gluconate gel can be applied topically if the patient is treated rapidly enough, that is before the HF has penetrated the skin. Diminished pain is the hallmark of effective treatment. Although direct injection of calcium gluconate into the burned area has long been advocated, this may not effectively neutralize HF and may cause skin necrosis. If irrigation and topical treatment with calcium has been ineffective, the patient should be treated with an intra-arterial infusion of calcium gluconate. Patients with extensive HF burns, and certainly patients with intra-arterial infusions, require close monitoring and should have frequent serum calcium checks.

SUMMARY

Successful treatment of the burned hand is challenging. Few burned areas have such a considerable effect on aesthetic and functional outcome of the patient. Proper treatment requires a multidisciplinary team approach for optimal outcomes. There are several controversial issues in the treatment of the burned hand, and they provide many opportunities for further research and analysis of current practices.

REFERENCES

1. Baker R, Jones S, Sanders C, et al. Degree of burn, location of burn, and length of hospital stay as predictor of psychosocial status and physical functioning. J Burn Care Rehabil 1996;17:327–33.
2. Anzarut A, Chen M, Shankowsky H, et al. Quality-of-life and outcome predictors following massive burn injury. Plast Reconstr Surg 2005;116(3):791–7.
3. Schneider JC, Holavanahalli R, Helm P, et al. Contractures in the burn injury part II: investigating joints of the hand. J Burn Care Res 2008;29(4):606–13.
4. Tredget EE. Management of the acutely burned upper extremity. Hand Clin 2000;16(2):187–203.
5. Engrav L, Heimbach DM, Reus J, et al. Early excision and grafting vs. nonoperative treatment of burns of indeterminant depth: a randomized prospective study. J Trauma 1983;23(11):1001–4.
6. American Burn Association. Burn center referral criteria. Available at: http://www.ameriburn.org/BurnCenterReferralCriteria.pdf. Accessed 2008.
7. American Burn Association. Advanced burn life support. Available at: http://www.ameriburn.org/ablsnow.php. Accessed 2008.
8. Luce EA. The acute and subacute management of the burned hand. Clin Plast Surg 2000;27(1):49–63.
9. Cartotto R. The burned hand: optimizing long term outcomes with standardized approach to acute and subacute care. Clin Plast Surg 2005;32(4):515–27.
10. Greenhalgh DG. Management of acute burn injuries of the upper extremity in the pediatric population. Hand Clin 2000;16(2):175–86.
11. Sheridan RL, Hurley J, Smith MA, et al. The acutely burned hand: management and outcomes based on a ten-year experience with 1047 acute hand burns. J Trauma 1995;38(3):406–11.
12. Smith MA, Munster AM, Spencer RJ. Burns of the hand and upper limb—a review. Burns 1998;24(6):493–505.
13. Kowalske K, Greenhalgh DG, Ward S. Hand burns. J Burn Care Res 2007;28(4):607–10.
14. Piccolo NS, Piccolo MS, Piccolo PD, et al. Escharotomies, fasciotomies and carpal tunnel release in burn patients-review of the literature and presentation of an algorithm for surgical decision making. Handchir Mikrochir Plast Chir 2007;39(3):161–7.
15. Cardoso R, Szabo RM. Wrist anatomy and surgical approaches. Orthop Clin North Am 2007;38(2):127–48.
16. Arnoldo B, Klein M, Gibran NS. Practice guidelines for the management of electrical injuries. J Burn Care Res 2006;27(4):439–47.
17. Wasiak J, Cleland H, Campbell F. Dressing for superficial and partial thickness burns. Cochrane Database Syst Rev. 2008 Oct;8(4):CD002106.

18. Salisbury RE. Reconstruction of the burned hand. Clin Plast Surg 2000;27(1):65–9.
19. Muangman P, Engrav LH, Heimbach D, et al. Complex wound management utilizing an artificial dermal matrix. Ann Plast Surg 2006;57(2):199–202.
20. Verolino P, Casoli V, Masia D, et al. A skin substitute (Integra) in a successful delayed reconstruction of a severe injured hand. Burns 2008;34(2):284–7.
21. Heimbach DM, Warden GD, Luterman A, et al. Multicenter postapproval clinical trial of Integra dermal regeneration template for burn treatment. J Burn Care Rehabil 2003;24(1):42–8.
22. Bhavsar D, Tenenhaus M. The use of acellular dermal matrix for coverage of exposed joint and extensor mechanism in thermally injured patients with few options. Eplasty 2008;8:e33.
23. Scott JR, Costa BA, Gibran NS, et al. Pediatric palm contact burns: a ten-year review. J Burn Care Res 2008;29(4):614–8.
24. Klein MB, Hunter S, Heimbach DM, et al. The Versajet water dissector: a new tool for tangential excision. J Burn Care Rehabil 2005;26(6):483–7.
25. Mann R, Gibran NS, Engrav LH, et al. Prospective trial of thick vs standard split-thickness skin grafts in burns of the hand. J Burn Care Rehabil 2001;22(6):390–2.
26. Foster K, Greenhalgh D, Gamelli RL, et al. Efficacy and safety of a fibrin sealant for adherence of autologous skin grafts to burn wounds: results of a phase 3 clinical study. J Burn Care Res 2008;29(2):293–303.
27. Davey RB. The use of an 'adhesive contact medium' (Hypafix) for split skin fixation: a 12-year review. Burns 1997;23(7–8):615–9.

Initial Management of Acute Pediatric Hand Burns

Tina L. Palmieri, MD, FACS, FCCM

KEYWORDS

- Burn evaluation • Hand injury • Pediatric • Treatment
- Outcomes

Children, because of their developmental imperative to explore their environment and their slow withdrawal reflex, are at high risk of sustaining burns. In fact, one-third of all US burn medical treatment visits involve children.[1] Hand burns are one of the leading causes of hand injury in children and can result in significant impairment of hand function.[2–7] Appropriate initial management of hand burns in children is imperative to optimize function and to minimize long-term scarring, and consequently, the American Burn Association advocates referral of pediatric hand burns to a verified burn center.[8] The philosophy "Do it right the first time" is particularly important in the care of pediatric hand burns, because early appropriate management can minimize tissue injury and improve long-term functional and psychosocial outcomes.[9]

Although hand function in adults and children depends on the integration of cognition with motor and sensory function, children and adults differ in the etiology, anatomy, and response to treatment of hand burns.[10–12] For example, preschool-aged children are developing fine motor skills and learning to interact with their environment. Injury during this developmental period can have an impact not just during healing but also on long-term hand function. Proper management of the child with burn injury is time consuming and resource intensive. A multidisciplinary approach, involving physicians, nurses, therapists, psychiatrists, and social support is needed to assure that the physical and psychosocial needs of the child and family are addressed.[13] The purpose of this article is to provide the reader with the foundation for appropriate initial evaluation and treatment of the child with hand burn injury, including etiology, anatomic considerations, assessment, wound management (initial operative and nonoperative), and rehabilitation issues.

ETIOLOGY

The cause of burn injury in children is influenced by the child's chronologic and developmental stage. Scald burns continue to constitute the vast majority of burns in children younger than 10 years; however, flame burns and contact burns predominate in young children with hand burns.[13] Certain patterns of injury are common. For example, dorsal hand burns are frequently caused by scald burns, whereas palm burns are frequently due to contact with a hot object, such as an iron or oven door (**Fig. 1**).[7,14] Iron burns involving the palm, in particular, are common in children younger than 2 years.[14] Friction burns to the hand and fingers from contact with a treadmill belt are increasingly being reported in the literature (**Fig. 2**).[15] These burns are due to the heat and tissue trauma generated by friction, and they often cause soft tissue loss or tendon injury. Electrical injuries are rare and most commonly involve contact with household current.

Approximately 10% of burn injuries cause suspicion of child abuse.[16,17] Several types of abuse typically result in hand burns: (1) immersion of the hand in hot water (resulting in a glovelike burn distribution), (2) forced contact with a hot object (such as an iron), or (3) flame burn from a cigarette lighter. A high index of suspicion of

Shriners Hospital for Children Northern California, University of California Davis, 2425 Stockton Boulevard, Suite 718, Sacramento, CA 95817, USA
E-mail address: tina.palmieri@ucdmc.ucdavis.edu

Hand Clin 25 (2009) 461–467
doi:10.1016/j.hcl.2009.06.006
0749-0712/09/$ – see front matter © 2009 Elsevier Inc. All rights reserved.

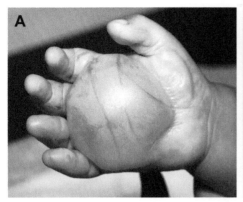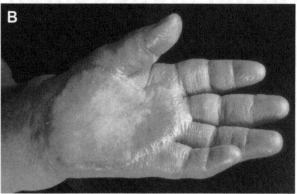

Fig. 1. Typical appearance of a palm burn of the hand before (*A*) and after (*B*) placement of a full-thickness skin graft.

abuse should be maintained and suspicious patterns referred to child protective services. In addition to medical care, the abused child will require psychological and social support. At times a child with a suspicious burn will need hospital admission until the details of the incident can be sorted out.

ANATOMY

The anatomy of a child's skin plays an important role in injury depth and healing as well as in the choice of treatment. The depth of a burn injury is related to several factors: (1) the length of time the skin is in contact with the heat source, (2) the temperature of the heat source, (3) the thickness of the skin, and (4) the blood supply to the skin. In response to injury, young children frequently "freeze" and do not quickly withdraw from heat, which leads to more prolonged contact with the heat source and more severe injury. Children have thinner skin than adults; hence, they sustain full-thickness burns at a lower temperature and after a shorter duration of contact than an adult.

However, toddlers have a thicker adipose layer between skin and tendon, which not only protects against injury but also facilitates the excision of the dorsal hand burn. Inguinal skin folds, which are common in small children, also provide a readily available source for full-thickness skin grafts.

The child's dorsal and palmar skin differ anatomically as well. The skin on the dorsal surface of the hand, although thin and flexible, also contains sebaceous glands, hair follicles, and pigment.[18] The palmar skin, unlike the dorsum of the hand, is thick, hairless, and has no pigment. As such, palmar skin requires longer contact with a higher temperature to result in a full-thickness burn. Due to the fibro-osseous tissue of the palmar surface of the hand and digits (such as pulp septa and Cleland ligaments), the palm has limited room for edema after burn injury, making it more susceptible to circulatory compromise. This is compounded by the dependent position and associated injuries of the arm.

Several areas of the child's hand pose special risks for long-term sequelae after burn injury. Injuries to the nail bed can result in nail deviation,

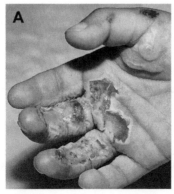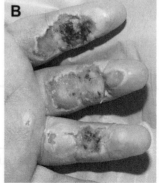

Fig. 2. Treadmill burns of the hand typically involve the volar surfaces of the fingers (*A*) and frequently extend to the level of the tendon (*B*).

cleft, loss, or discoloration and affect hand function adversely.[19] The extensor tendons of the proximal interphalangeal joint (PIP) are another vulnerable area. The central slip of the extensor tendon inserts into the PIP, while two lateral bands continue distally to the base of the phalanx. Disruption of this mechanism results in the boutonnière deformity. Finally, the hypermobility of the metacarpophalangeal joint of the fifth finger puts it at risk of a boutonnière deformity months after excision and grafting.[20]

HISTORY OF HAND BURN TREATMENT

The treatment of hand burns has varied with time. Management before the twentieth century, before the advent of burn centers, involved the use of creams, salves, and home remedies until the eschar separated or the wound healed.[21] The outcome depended on the wound depth: (1) A superficial wound would heal without a scar; (2) A deep partial-thickness wound would heal after 2 to 4 weeks, with a thickened scar and decreased joint motion (if the burn extended over a joint); and (3) A deep full-thickness burn would result in marked deformity, chronic open wound, or amputation. A variety of treatments were advocated in the early 1900s, including petroleum gauze, wax, and tannic acid.[22–24] Although aggressive early surgical excision and range of motion were introduced in the 1940s, the major challenge to burn care at that time was survival, and treatment of hand burns assumed a less important role.[25,26] It was not until the 1970s that early excision of hand burns was shown to decrease the need for future reconstructive surgery and improve outcomes.[27–29] Early excision and grafting of full-thickness burns with aggressive therapy remain the mainstay of treatment today.

EVALUATION AND MANAGEMENT OF THE BURNED HAND

As with the evaluation of any patient with traumatic injury, life-threatening injuries precede the hand injury during evaluation. The history of the injury will provide clues to potential associated trauma (crush injury or motor vehicle crash) or possible child abuse. The parent and child, if developmental stage allows, should be interviewed regarding the circumstances of the injury. The type of burn (flame, scald, or contact), duration of contact with heat, and prior hand injuries should be recorded. Radiographs are generally unnecessary unless there is associated traumatic injury. Extent and depth of the burn should be assessed. Burn extent can be estimated in two ways: (1)

using the notion that the patient's palm (including fingers) is 1% of the body, or (2) using the Lund-Browder chart, which provides body surface area estimates based on age. Circumferential burns of the hand and/or upper extremity should be noted. Burn depth determination in the hand can be somewhat challenging, especially in the presence of bullae. In general, the tenets of hand burn care in children are: (1) Promote a wound-healing environment, (2) Maintain circulation, (3) Prevent infection, (4) Obtain wound closure, and (5) Maintain motion. Appropriate initial wound care relies on knowledge of the pathophysiology of burn wounds.

Promote a Wound-Healing Environment

Pathophysiologically, the burn wound contains three different zones of injury: coagulation, stasis, and hyperemia. These zones are dynamic and are influenced by tissue circulation and wound care. The zone of coagulation represents an area of irretrievable injury, that is, tissue is damaged beyond repair. The zone of hyperemia is a mild injury that will heal spontaneously within 7 to 10 days. The zone of stasis is the area that has significant cell injury, but cells are initially viable. Appropriate wound management will avert further injury, whereas inappropriate management or lack of circulation will increase the damage. The goal of initial wound care is thus to minimize the conversion of the zone of stasis to the zone of coagulation; this is done by optimizing the environment for healing.

First, all loose debris and broken blisters should be debrided from the wound, as they are a nidus for infection. In general, palm blisters can be left intact; however, if the blister compromises circulation or impedes range of motion, it may require debridement. Any blister 2 cm or less in height on the palm, as a rule, can be left intact without causing circulatory compromise. Once the blister ruptures, however, the loose tissue should be debrided. Intact blisters should be wrapped in dry dressings; topical antimicrobials are ineffective and will only macerate the blister. Cleansing and application of topical antimicrobials are appropriate after the blister has ruptured. Dressing changes should be performed at least daily and the wound reevaluated by a medical professional weekly until healed.

Maintain Circulation

Maintaining circulation in the burned hand is the next priority. Patients with major burns (>20% of total body surface area) should receive appropriate intravenous resuscitation. Hand burns should be elevated and dressings placed loosely to avoid circulatory compromise. Escharotomy may be necessary if the patient has marked perfusion abnormality as evidenced by decreasing temperature, delayed capillary refill, decreased pulsatile perfusion of the palmar arch, increasing pain, and increasing turgor of hand compartments. Care should be taken to ensure that vascular compromise of the hand is not due to compartment syndrome of the arm or forearm.

Hand escharotomy is rarely necessary after burn injury, and it risks not only blood loss but also injury to underlying structures. Hand escharotomy should only be performed by a trained burn surgeon or hand surgeon. After intravenous sedation is administered, electrocautery is used to incise through burn eschar to pliable nonconstricting tissue or fat. For the arm, escharotomies are performed along the medial and lateral aspects of the extremity with the arm supinated so as to avoid vital structures. In the hand, the compartments are released with 2 to 3 longitudinal dorsal incisions on the dorsal aspect between tendons.[30] Digital escharotomies are of questionable benefit. If needed, they are performed along the lateral and medial aspects of the fingers and should be above the skin crease formed when the finger is bent at the distal interphalangeal joint to avoid neurovascular injury. Regardless, circulation should be reassessed frequently after the performance of escharotomies. If the hand shows evidence of continuing circulatory compromise, fasciotomy in the operating room by a qualified hand surgeon may be necessary.

Prevent Infection

Infection of the burned hand is most readily prevented by early cleansing of the wound with an antimicrobial soap, removing loose tissue, and rinsing with water. If blisters remain intact, no topical antimicrobial therapy is necessary. However, once blisters rupture, debridement of the tissue and placement of a topical antimicrobial is generally advisable. A partial-thickness wound, which is classically pink, moist, and painful, will heal in less than 2 weeks and can be treated with topical bacitracin and Adaptic Dressing (Johnson and Johnson, New Brunswick, New Jersey) or petroleum gauze such as Xeroform (Coridan Health, St Louis, Missouri) once or twice daily. Silver sulfadiazine should be reserved for obvious third-degree burns because, although it has broader antimicrobial coverage, it is harder to clean and impedes wound healing.[31] Other potential partial-thickness dressings include

Biobrane (Smith and Nephew, Manhattan, New York), Glucan (Beta Glucan, Brennan, St. Paul, Minnesota), and Neosporin (Johnson and Johnson, New Brunswick, New Jersey) (small wounds).[32,33] Other topical agents for full-thickness wounds include mafenide acetate (reserved for ears and invasive infections), silver nitrate solution (causes skin discoloration), and silver-containing dressings.

Obtain Wound Closure

The goal of burn wound treatment is to obtain wound coverage, with autologous tissue strong and pliable enough to allow maximal hand function. The need for surgical intervention is dictated by the depth and location of the wound. Partial-thickness burns that heal within 2 weeks do not, in general, require grafting and will not develop significant scarring. These wounds should be managed in a moist environment to encourage epithelialization.[34] Skin grafting should be considered for virtually all deep partial-thickness burns that do not heal within 2 weeks and for full-thickness hand burns.[13,35,36]

When considering surgical intervention, the simplest technique that allows wound closure without compromising function should be used. Operative intervention should occur within 3 days of the initial burn in cases of deep partial- and full-thickness hand burns. Early excision not only prevents infection but also facilitates wound excision, as the subeschar edema creates a natural tissue plane and the burn wound has not been degraded. The burn eschar should be excised tangentially using a Goulian knife. Use of a tourniquet decreases blood loss and improves visualization of depth of excision. After tourniquet deflation, the wound is inspected for adequacy of excision, and hemostasis is obtained.

The two most frequently used skin graft techniques are full-thickness grafts (incorporating all layers of the skin and requiring closure) or split-thickness grafts (tangential shaving of skin at the dermal-epidermal junction that will heal with proper wound care). Split-thickness skin grafts are often required on the dorsum of the hand due to the increased width and length of the dorsal finger surface. Split-thickness grafts have a higher engraftment rate, especially on marginal wound beds. However, split-thickness skin grafts also have greater contraction, more scarring, less sensation, and potential for worse cosmetic outcomes than full-thickness grafts. Full-thickness skin grafts are particularly apropos for the palm, as a graft can usually be obtained from the child's inguinal crease to cover the entire surface of the palm (see **Fig. 1**B).[7] Full-thickness grafts are limited by availability of donor sites and, because inguinal skin has pigmentation, will be darker than the adjacent unburned palm skin. Sheet-split or full-thickness skin grafts should be used whenever possible, to maximize cosmetic and functional outcomes. If sheet skin grafts are used, the burn excision should include the dermal elements (ie, extend to the level of fat) to avoid the formation of inclusion cysts after engraftment. Meshed grafts heal by scarring of the interstices, which leaves a visible meshed pattern that can increase contracture formation. However, use of sheet grafts is contingent on skin availability and adequacy of the wound bed. It may be impractical to use sheet grafts for children with full-thickness burns covering more than 90% of total body surface area in which maximizing coverage is a life-saving maneuver. Allograft, xenograft, or Integra (Integra LifeSciences, Plainsboro, New Jersey) may be used as temporary coverage when an adequate donor site for hand grafts is not available.

Optimal donor-site location for split-thickness skin grafts differs between adults and children. In children, there is decreased long-term donor-site scarring on the back, and there is no difference in infection rate, pigmentation, or blistering compared with the thigh.[37] Hence, the back is the donor site of choice for split-thickness skin grafts in children. An additional adjunct for use in hand burns is the 6-inch dermatome, which can eliminate midline seams in the graft. This dermatome is particularly suited to the wide, flat surface of the back. Full-thickness skin grafts are usually obtained from the inguinal crease or the abdomen.

Fourth-degree burns (involving tendon, joint, muscle, and bone), often lead to functional impairment. Initially, autologous or cadaveric skin grafts can be used to delineate tissue viability. In cases of digit joint instability, Kirschner wires can be inserted axially to immobilize the joint in a position of function until autografting is complete. Approximately 25% of patients treated with wire fixation will have significant restriction in activities of daily living.[13] Flaps (either regional or free) may be required in the case of extensive fourth-degree injury involving multiple fingers. Amputation should only be performed for digits that are mummified or unsalvageable.

Maintain Motion

Maintaining range of motion in the child with hand burn injury is important to prevent future contractures. For patients with partial-thickness burns, parents should be instructed on extremity range-of-motion exercises for the child and in encouraging the child to use the hand during play. Splints may be needed to maintain the hand in a functional position. As a rule, hand splints involve 20° of wrist extension, 70° to 90° metacarpophalangeal joint flexion, and extension of the interphalangeal joint. After skin grafting, passive range of motion should be initiated as soon as grafts are stable (generally 5–7 days postgrafting). Strength, range of motion, and coordination of movement patterns should be monitored and encouraged by a hand therapist. Pressure garments can be helpful in decreasing edema and facilitating restoration of motion. However, pressure garments need to be closely monitored and modified as the child grows. In general, a pressure garment for a child will need modification every 3 to 4 months. Silicon sheeting may be helpful in decreasing scar prominence. Hand splints or molds may be needed to maintain the hand in the neutral position at night.

LONG-TERM ISSUES IN PEDIATRIC HAND BURNS

Although children can regain full hand function after third-degree hand burns, vigilance is needed to address contracture and scar formation and problems in range of motion. Range of motion and strength, as mentioned earlier, are vital components in long-term hand therapy. Despite appropriate therapy, however, children can develop scar contractures due to their growth. Contractures tend to form at sites of graft failure, joints, and web spaces. Contracture release is indicated in any hand with a burn scar contracture that significantly impedes hand function despite appropriate splinting, stretching, and therapy. Early surgical burn scar contracture release, using the reconstruction ladder, is indicated for contractures that threaten joint function or hand growth. Waiting for a scar to mature for 6 to 12 months can result in permanent deformities. However, care needs to be taken that early release is done only after failure of nonoperative therapies and in patients and families who are committed to participating in postoperative hand therapy.[38]

A complete discussion of hand burn reconstruction is beyond the scope of this article. Several techniques are commonly used in hand reconstruction, including Z-plasty, double-opposing Z-plasty, local flaps, release and full- or split-thickness skin grafts, and free flaps. Web space contractures can often be addressed using either a double-opposing Z-plasty or a full-thickness graft. Palm contractures frequently require release and full-thickness skin grafting. Hand therapy postreconstructive procedure is vital; otherwise, hand function is likely to be compromised.

SUMMARY

Hand burns in children are a frequent and potentially devastating injury and should be cared for in centers with the necessary resources and experience to address all aspects of care. Appropriate initial evaluation and treatment and proper long-term management using a multidisciplinary team will optimize the functional outcomes of children with hand burns.

REFERENCES

1. Duffy BJ, McLaughlin PM, Eichelberger MR. Assessment, triage, and early management of burns in children. Clin Pediatr Emerg Med 2006;7:82–93.
2. Exner CE. Remediation of hand skill problems in children. In: Henderson A, Pehoski C, editors. Hand function in the child: foundations for remediation. St. Louis (MO): Mosby; 1995. p. 197–222.
3. Zamboni WA, Cassidy M, Eriksson E, et al. Hand burns in children under 5 years of age. Burns Incl Therm Inj 1987;13(6):476–83.
4. Johnson CF, Kaufman KL, Callendar C, et al. The hand as a target organ in child abuse. Clin Pediatr (Phila) 1990;29(2):66–72.
5. Agran PF, Anderson C, Winn D, et al. Rates of pediatric injury by 3-month intervals for children 0 to 3 years of age. Pediatrics 2003;111:e683–92.
6. Chait LA. Treatment of contact burns of the palm in children. S Afr Med J 1975;49:1839–42.
7. Pham TN, Hanley C, Palmieri TL, et al. Results of early excision and full-thickness grafting of deep palm burns in children. J Burn Care Rehabil 2001;22:54–7.
8. American College of Surgeons. Guidelines for the operation of Burn Centers. In: Resources for optimal care of the injured patient. Committee on Trauma; 2006. p. 79–86.
9. Greenhalgh DG. Management of acute burn injuries of the upper extremity in the pediatric population. Hand Clin 2000;16:175–86.
10. Case-Smith J. Grasp, release, and bimanual skills in the first two years of life. In: Henderson A, Pehoski C, editors. Hand function in the child: foundations for remediation. St. Louis (MO): Mosby; 1995. p. 113–36.
11. Case-Smith J. The relationships among sensorimotor components, fine motor skill, and functional performance in preschool children. Am J Occup Ther 1995;49(7):645–52.
12. Clarke HM, Wittpenn GP, McLeod AM, et al. Acute management of pediatric hand burns. Hand Clin 1990;6:221–32.
13. Sheridan RL, Baryza MJ, Pessina MA, et al. Acute hand burn in children: management and long-term outcome based on a 10-year experience with 698 injured hands. Ann Surg 1999;229:558–64.
14. Brown RL, Greenhalgh DG, Warden GD. Iron burns to the hand in the young pediatric patient: a problem in prevention. J Burn Care Rehabil 1997;18:279–82.
15. Carman C, Chang B. Treadmill injuries to the upper extremity in pediatric patients. Ann Plast Surg 2001; 47:15–9.
16. Showers J, Garrison KM. Burn abuse: a four-year study. J Trauma 1988;28:1581–3.
17. Hummel RP, Greenhalgh DG, Barthel PP, et al. Outcome and socioeconomic aspects of suspected child abuse scald burns. J Burn Care Rehabil 1993; 14:121–6.
18. Feldmann ME, Evans J, O SJ. Early management of the burned pediatric hand. J Craniofac Surg 2008; 19:942–50.
19. Spauwen PH, Brown IF, Sauer EW, et al. Management of fingernail deformities after thermal injury. Scand J Plast Reconstr Surg Hand Surg 1987;21: 253–5.
20. Simpson RL, Flaherty ME. The burned small finger. Clin Plast Surg 1992;19:673–82.
21. Cockshott WP. The history of the treatment of burns. Surg Gynecol Obstet 1956;102:116.
22. Sherman W. The paraffin wax or closed method of treatment of burns. Surg Gynecol Obstet 1918;26: 450.
23. Allen HS. Treatment of superficial injuries and burns of the hand. JAMA 1941;116:1370.
24. Bunnell S. Reconstructive surgery of the hand. Surg Gynecol Obstet 1924;39:259.
25. Cope O, Langohr JL, Moore FD, et al. Expeditious care of full-thickness burn wound by surgical excision and grafting. Ann Surg 1947;125:1.
26. McCorkle HJ, Silvani H. Selection of the time for grafting of skin to extensive defects resulting from deep thermal burns. Ann Surg 1945;121:285–90.
27. Burke JF, Bondoc CC, Quinby WC Jr, et al. Primary surgical management of the deeply burned hand. J Trauma 1976;16:593–8.
28. Bondoc CC, Quinby WC, Burke JF. Primary surgical management of the deeply burned hand in children. J Pediatr Surg 1976;11:355–62.
29. Frist W, Ackroyd F, Burke J, et al. Long-term functional results of selective treatment of hand burns. Am J Surg 1985;149:516–21.
30. Smith MA, Munster AM, Spence RJ. Burns of the hand and upper limb-a review. Burns 1998;24: 493–505.
31. Palmieri TL, Greenhalgh DG. Topical treatment of pediatric patients with burns: a practical guide. Am J Clin Dermatol 2002;3:529–34.
32. Delatte SJ, Evans J, Hebra A, et al. Effectiveness of beta-glucan collagen for treatment of partial-thickness burns in children. J Pediatr Surg 2001;36: 113–8.
33. Barret JP, Dziewulski P, Ramzy PI, et al. Biobrane versus 1% silver sulfadiazine in second-degree

pediatric burns. Plast Reconstr Surg 2000;105: 62–5.

34. Rovee DT, Kurowsky CA, Labun J. Local wound environment and epidermal healing. Mitotic response. Arch Dermatol 1972;106:330–4.

35. Sheridan, Salisbury RE, Wright P. Evaluation of early excision of dorsal burns of the hand. Plast Reconstr Surg 1982;69:670–5.

36. Robson MC, Smith DJ Jr, VanderZee AJ, et al. Making the burned hand functional. Clin Plast Surg 1992;19:663–71.

37. Greenhalgh DG, Barthel PP, Warden GD. Comparison of back versus thigh donor sites in pediatric patients with burns. J Burn Care Rehabil 1993;14:21–5.

38. Schwarz RJ. Management of postburn contractures of the upper extremity. J Burn Care Res 2007;28: 212–9.

The Diagnosis and Management of Electrical Injuries

Brett D. Arnoldo, MD*, Gary F. Purdue, MD

KEYWORDS

- Electrical burns • Fasciotomy • Rhabdomyolysis
- ECG monitoring

Electricity is a ubiquitous and indispensable part of modern civilization. Electrical burns typically comprise a small percentage of total admissions to major burn centers; reportedly about 5%.[1,2] These injuries are, however, the most devastating of all thermal injuries on a size-for-size basis, usually involving both skin and deeper tissues. They affect primarily young, working men, and are the most frequent cause of amputations within the burn service.[3,4] These injuries account for nearly 6% of all occupational fatalities annually.[5]

Electrical injuries have several unique acute manifestations that differ from other thermal injuries and require expertise in management. Decisions must be made about cardiac monitoring, emergent exploration and decompression of extremity compartments, and the treatment of myoglobinuria. These decisions, which are made in the acute setting, in addition to management decisions common to all thermal injuries, have profound effects on outcomes. Even with state-of-the-art care in an American Burn Association verified burn center, morbidity, length of hospital stay, and number of operations on electrical injuries are higher than expected, based on burn size.[4]

PATHOPHYSIOLOGY

Electrical injury severity is determined by voltage (E), current (amperage; I), current type (alternating or direct), path of current flow, duration of contact, resistance at the point of contact, and individual susceptibility. Clinically the only factors that are easily defined are voltage and type of current. Electrical burns are arbitrarily divided into high voltage ($\geq$ 1000 V) and low voltage (< 1000 V). Voltage is usually known by the injured individual, coworkers, or bystanders, or is determined by the environment in which the burn occurs. Most high-voltage injuries occur in workers on the job so the voltage is known. The United States, Canadian, and Mexican domestic power grids operate on alternating current (AC) at 120 V, thus injuries that occur indoors in North America are almost exclusively low-voltage AC (excepting some specialized industrial settings). Our AC power system operates at 60 Hz. AC at 60 Hz (or 60 cycles per second), reverses polarity 120 times per second. With one half of the time spent positive with respect to ground and one half spent negative, the verbiage "entrance" and "exit" wounds should be abandoned. These wounds should be referred to as "contact points." In addition, the injury itself should not be referred to as an electrocution. The Merriam-Webster definition of "electrocution" is (1) to execute by electricity; (2) to kill by electric shock.[6] Efforts to quantify the amount of current in the clinical setting will not be fruitful as current varies in a reciprocal fashion with resistance according to Ohm's law: Current (I) = Voltage (E)/Resistance (R).

Resistance varies continuously with time, initially dropping slowly, then much more rapidly until arcing occurs at the contact sites. Resistance then rises to infinity and current flow ceases.[7] Temperature increase parallels changes in amperage with tissue temperature being a critical

Department of Surgery, University of Texas Southwestern Medical Center, 5323 Harry Hines Blvd., Dallas, TX 75390-9158, USA
* Corresponding author.
E-mail address: brett.arnoldo@utsouthwestern.edu (B.D. Arnoldo).

Hand Clin 25 (2009) 469–479
doi:10.1016/j.hcl.2009.06.001

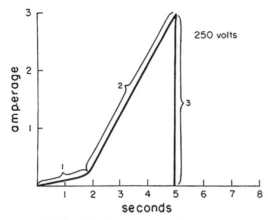

Fig. 1. Relationship of amperage to time.

factor in the magnitude of tissue damage (**Figs. 1 and 2**).[7]

The path of current flow has impact on patient complications and survival. However, accurate description is difficult at best. A vertical pathway parallel to the axis of the body is the most dangerous in that it involves all the organs of the body, including the conducting system of the heart, the respiratory muscles, and the central nervous system (CNS). A horizontal pathway from hand to hand may still be fatal as it can involve the heart respiratory musculature and the CNS. A pathway through the lower portions of the body would be less likely to be lethal.[8] Determination of the current pathway is at best a clinical guess.

AC causes tetanic muscle contraction, which may either throw victims away from contact or draw them into continued contact with the electrical source, the latter being more common given our propensity to grasp at objects and the greater strength in our forearm flexors relative to extensors. This effect is the often described "no-let-go" phenomenon. Altered levels of consciousness, reported in about half of high-voltage

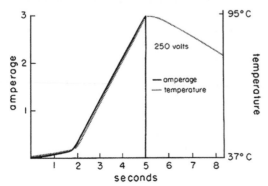

Fig. 2. Relationship of amperage, temperature, and time.

victims, also contribute to the prolonged periods of contact.[9]

Resistance at the point of contact varies from very low values for sweat-soaked hands or skin in the summer to more than 100,000 ohms for heavily calloused hands during dry winter months. Individual susceptibility is a nonquantifiable term used to explain why two or more individuals exposed to the same situation have extremely varied injuries. Tissue resistance from lowest to highest is nerve, blood vessels, muscle, skin, tendon, fat, and bone. Once the resistance of the skin is overcome, current flow through tissue is theoretically distributed proportional to resistance, with tissue having the highest resistance generating the most heat. However, in the animal model the internal tissue acts as a single uniform resistance and not as a compendium of multiple resistors (ie, a volume conductor).[7] Deep tissue seems to retain heat so that periosseous tissues, especially between two bones, often sustain a more severe injury than more superficial tissue. The associated macro- and microscopic vascular injury seems to occur nearly immediately and is not reversible.[10]

The burn injury caused by electricity may be categorized as: (1) true electrical injury caused by current flow against tissue resistance causing heating of tissue; (2) direct thermal burn from the heat of arcing that is caused when high-voltage current passes through the air; and (3) thermal burn from ignited clothes or surroundings. Electricity arcs at temperatures of up to 4000°C, creating a flash-type injury[11] most commonly seen in electricians working with metal objects close to an electrical source. When occurring without actual current injury, these injuries are treated in the same manner as any flash burn.

The tissue injury in electrical burns seems to be a combination of thermal and nonthermal mechanisms. Electricity flows through tissue and generates power (heat) according to Joule's law:

$$Power(J, Joule) = I^2(Current) \times R(Resistance)$$

Joule heating is in simple terms the frying of tissue. In more scientific terms it is the transfer of energy that occurs when charged particles lose energy to the tissues in the form of heat. If enough heat is generated, the tissue heats to supraphysiologic temperatures causing denaturation of macromolecules, which is usually irreversible.[12] Electroporation refers to the formation of aqueous pores in lipid bilayers exposed to a supraphysiologic electric field. The applied electric field alters the transmembrane potential, with muscle fibers and nerves being the most susceptible. Subsequent pore formation likely allows calcium influx into the cytoplasm thereby triggering apoptosis and cell death. Electroporation can therefore induce cell necrosis in the absence of joule heating.[13–15] Transmembrane protein molecules contain polar amino acid residues that can change orientation in an electric field. This effect, known as electroconformational protein degradation, may be irreversible and form yet another mechanism of nonthermal injury.[16]

Severity of injury is proportional to the cross-sectional area of tissue able to carry current. Thus the most severe injuries are seen at the wrists and ankles, with decreasing severity proximally. The extremities are the most frequently injured body parts, with the upper extremity predominating.[4]

ACUTE CARE

Initial evaluation follows the protocols established by the American College of Surgeons Advanced Trauma Life Support (ATLS) and the American Burn Association as part of the Advanced Burn Life Support (ABLS) courses. Protection of the field team is a first priority and responders must ensure that electrical power at the scene is disconnected before proceeding to handle the patient. The ABCDE primary survey priorities, followed by the secondary survey, are as outlined in the aforementioned courses. Approximately 15% of electrical burn victims sustain traumatic injuries in addition to their burn, a rate nearly double that of other burn patients. Most of these injuries are caused by falls from a height or being thrown against an object, with some resulting from tetanic muscle contractions associated with the electrical shock; forces strong enough to cause compression fractures.[17] The examiner needs to maintain vigilance and not be distracted by the often dramatic presentation of these injuries.

FLUID RESUSCITATION AND HEMOCHROMAGENS

Estimates of fluid requirements are a standard part of the resuscitation phase of the thermally injured patient. The Parkland (Baxter) formula[18] is the most commonly used of these estimates. The deep tissue injury associated with high-voltage electrical injuries renders this and other formulas based on body surface area burned inaccurate, except to establish a minimum volume required. In the absence of gross urinary pigmentation the goal of resuscitation is to maintain normal vital signs and a urine output of 30 to 50 mL/h (or 0.5 mL/kg) with Ringer lactate. Urine output should

be followed hourly and changes made in the intravenous (IV) fluid rate generally in increments of 10% to 20% of the current rate. The administration of fluid boluses in burn patients is generally discouraged in all but the direst of circumstances; fluid boluses in this patient population increase third space losses.

The presence of gross pigmenturia (darker than light pink) (**Fig. 3**) in a patient with an electrical burn indicates significant muscle damage. The responsible pigments are myoglobin, secondary to rhabdomyolysis, and free hemoglobin, from lysed red blood cells. Gross pigmenturia is diagnosed visually and confirmed positive on dipstick test for blood and negative on microscopy for red blood cells. Confirmatory urine myoglobin assay is unnecessary and adds little to management. As with all burn trauma patients, associated injuries such as bladder or kidney injuries must be considered.

Myoglobin plays a dominant role in the pathogenesis of rhabdomyolysis-induced acute renal failure. The mechanisms involved include: (1) renal constriction and ischemia, (2) myoglobin cast formation in the distal convoluted tubule, and (3) direct cytotoxic action of myoglobin on epithelial cells of the proximal convoluted tubules.[19–22] Several methods have been proposed in the treatment of rhabdomyolysis and myoglobinuria. However, the most important component is adequate fluid resuscitation and high urine output. In this setting the fluid rate should be titrated to maintain a urine output of approximately 100 mL/h until the urine visually appears clear. Several methods to enhance renal clearance of myoglobin have been proposed, including osmotic diuresis with mannitol and alkalinization of the urine.[23] These adjuncts are not supported by level I evidence and represent individual centers' practices.[24,25] A recent retrospective study in a large

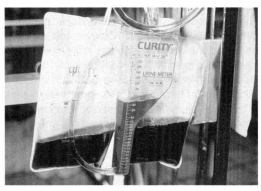

Fig. 3. The appearance of pigmented urine signifying muscle damage.

trauma center showed no differences in outcome with the addition of bicarbonate and mannitol in patients with rhabdomyolysis.[26] The authors, however, use a protocol of 2 ampules of sodium bicarbonate and 25 grams of mannitol, both given as an IV push in the treatment of grossly pigmented urine. The authors have had a zero incidence of acute renal failure in more than 270 consecutive patients with grossly visible urinary pigment. Patients who do not clear their urine may require repeat doses of bicarbonate and mannitol. These patients need to be evaluated for ongoing ischemia and muscle necrosis, and will often require surgical intervention for emergent compartment decompression or amputation. Additional evidence of ongoing muscle ischemia or myonecrosis requiring surgical intervention is increasing serum creatine kinase isoenzymes. The authors do not routinely obtain and follow isoenzymes for this purpose, as muscle necrosis requiring surgical intervention is usually clinically obvious and this additional laboratory value is unnecessary in making the diagnosis.

ELECTROCARDIOGRAPHIC MONITORING

Although ventricular fibrillation is the most common cause a death at the scene of injury, virtually any cardiac dysrhythmias can be precipitated by an electrical injury. Dysrhythmias are treated using the same indications and modalities as for medical causes. In the authors' experience, new onset atrial fibrillation has been the most common dysrhythmia seen in patients reaching the hospital alive. All have responded to medical management. An electrocardiogram (ECG) should be performed in all patients who sustain electrical injuries (high and low voltage). Cardiac monitoring is indicated for: (1) ECG abnormalities, (2) cardiac dysrhythmia during transport or in the emergency room, (3) documented cardiac arrest, (4) loss of consciousness, and (5) patients with other standard indications (total body surface area burn [TBSA] and so forth). The duration of cardiac monitoring is generally between 24 and 48 hours; however, this is based on scant data.[27] Most patients with low-voltage injury and no indication for monitoring can be safely discharged from the emergency room. The institutional policy of the authors is to apply these criteria to the high-voltage injuries based on their own published data, although this is not universally accepted in all institutions. Other recent reports do, however, suggest that all cardiac irregularities are evident either on admission to the emergency room or within several hours of hospitalization, and that cardiac monitoring in these patients may not be indicated.[28–30]

Direct myocardial injury may also result. These injuries behave more like traumatic myocardial contusion than true myocardial infarction, not having the hemodynamic or recurrence consequences of atherosclerotic myocardial infarctions. Housinger and colleagues have shown that creatine kinase (CK) and MB-creatine kinase (CK-MB) levels are poor indicators of myocardial injury in the absence of ECG findings of myocardial damage, especially in the presence of significant skeletal muscle injury.[31–33] Given the paucity of evidence supporting the utility of CK-MB levels, this laboratory value should not be used as a diagnostic criterion for cardiac injury after electrical injury. The utility of troponin levels in these patients for the determination of cardiac injury is unclear.

COMPARTMENT SYNDROME

Patients with high-voltage electrical injuries are at risk for deep tissue damage and compartment syndrome. The adage "what you see is what you get" seems to hold true when applied to low-voltage injuries. The clinician must be alert to the possibility of more extensive injury in high-voltage injuries, however (**Figs. 4** and **5**). Tight compartments and muscle necrosis may develop during the first 48 hours post injury. Damaged muscle, swelling within the investing fascia of the extremity, may increase pressure to the point at which muscle blood flow is compromised. Loss of pulses is one of the last signs of compartment syndrome. A high index of suspicion is paramount to early diagnosis (either by serial examinations or compartment pressures). Previously a very aggressive approach has been recommended given the morbidity associated with missed injury. This approach often included the recommendation of early (within 24 hours post burn) exploration and debridement.[34–37] Amputation rates were generally reported to be in the 35% to 40% range in

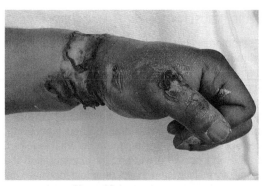

Fig. 4. Contracted hand with deep contact point at wrist.

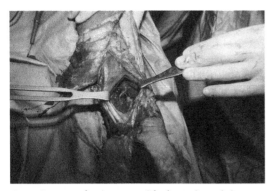

Fig. 5. Forearm fasciotomy with deep tissue injury.

most of these series. Indications for surgery in a recent evidence-based guideline article were (1) progressive neurologic dysfunction, (2) vascular compromise, (3) increased compartment pressure, and (4) systemic clinical deterioration from suspected ongoing myonecrosis.[27] Patients not meeting these indications may be debrided on the third to fifth postinjury day.[38] The diagnosis of compartment syndrome may be made clinically with or without adjunctive studies, such as measured compartment pressures greater than 30 mm Hg. The authors have found that measuring compartment pressures is unnecessary for diagnosis. Most commonly the decision to explore and decompress can be confidently made in the emergency department at the time of initial assessment. Patients who are not diagnosed with compartment syndrome in the emergency department but go on to develop this complication later (at 24–48 hours), generally had findings at initial assessment that were missed, or bigger cutaneous burns and a large fluid requirement. These are not subtle injuries. Elevated CK levels have been correlated with the extent of muscle damage, with investigators advocating early decompression and aggressive management for strongly elevated CK levels.[39] In the authors' experience these adjunctive studies do not often add much to the clinical picture that is not already obvious based on physical examination. Doppler flowmetry may be used as an adjunct in the diagnosis of these injuries. Although the Doppler signal from the distal arteries and palmar arch is a more sensitive indicator of perfusion than clinical palpation in circumferential burns, it should not be relied on as a sole indicator of deep tissue viability and the need for escharotomies or fasciotomy in electrical injuries.[40,41]

Four compartment fasciotomies of the lower leg are the standard of care, and this operation is well within the purview of the general surgeon. Upper extremity compartment syndrome, however, is not a clinical entity seen often by most general

surgeons and is yet one more reason why electrical injuries require referral to a burn center.

Operative intervention should proceed on an emergent basis and requires general anesthesia. Fluid resuscitation should occur simultaneously with surgery, requiring an experienced team approach and good communication.

The forearm fasciotomies must decompress the flexor (volar) compartment, the mobile wad (brachioradialis, extensor carpi radialis longus, and brevis), and the extensor (dorsal) compartment. This maneuver requires two separate incisions. A carpal tunnel release is included in the volar release as well in all but the rarest of patients. The authors prefer the lazy-S incision for the volar surface. The incision originates on the medial aspect of the arm 1 to 2 cm proximal to the medial epicondyle. The incision is extended obliquely across the antecubital fossa to reach the volar aspect of the mobile wad and is continued distally and curving ulnarly, reaching the midline at approximately the junction of the middle and distal thirds of the forearm. The incision is extended to the wrist just ulnar to the palmaris longus tendon, and is then carried across the wrist at an angle and extended into the mid palm. It should be carried no further radially than the mid axis of the ring finger. The subcutaneous tissue is incised to expose the deep fascia, which is examined, incised, and the muscles mobilized as necessary.[42–45] Potential areas of median nerve compression occur at the bicipital aponeurosis, the pronator teres, the deep fascial surface of the flexor digitorum superficialis, and the carpal tunnel. All but the carpal tunnel are released with relative ease through the lazy-S incision. The simplest method for carpal tunnel release uses straight scissors, inserting the open jaw under the transverse carpal ligament (while remaining ulnar to the palmaris longus tendon), and then simply pushing across the ligament. This maneuver is not for the inexperienced but an adequate release is ensured with this technique.

The extensor compartment is simpler and requires a straight longitudinal incision over the dorsal surface of the forearm. The incision begins 1 to 2 cm lateral and 2 cm distal to the lateral epicondyle, and is extended distally toward the midline of the wrist for 8 to 10 cm in length. Debridement of clearly necrotic nonviable muscle may proceed at this initial operation. A conservative approach is taken with tissue of questionable viability. Amputation at initial operation is reserved for mummified, contracted extremities. The initial operation is followed by a second look at 24 to 48 hours, with debridement or amputation and earliest possible closure. Coverage of the ensuing wound is with a biologic dressing such as porcine heterograft and the extremity is kept elevated to hasten resolution of edema. Fasciotomy wound closure is facilitated by use of traction on the affected skin edges by carefully placed sutures or vessel loop tensioning.[46] Wounds with associated skin and muscle loss often require skin grafting; however, closure can often be facilitated with a V.A.C. dressing.

WOUND CARE

Wound care of burned skin proceeds according to good practice guidelines as outlined in ABLS. The thick contact points are best treated with mefanide acetate (Sulfamylon) for good broad-spectrum coverage and excellent eschar penetration. Silver sulfadiazine topical coverage is typically used for the flash/flame component of the injury.

Surgical excision of wounds is typically begun 2 to 3 days post burn either as a second-look operation following fasciotomy or as the first procedure in patients not requiring fasciotomy. All obvious necrotic tissue is removed, while tissues of questionable viability are retained and reevaluated every 2 to 3 days until wound closure can be achieved. A conservative course of tissue removal and wound closure with a combination skin grafts or flaps for soft tissue coverage gives the best functional results. Progression of tissue necrosis that is observed clinically in these wounds is the guiding principle to conservative serial debridement. Studies of these injuries, however, have failed to support the notion of progressive ischemia secondary to electrically induced endothelial damage. In serial arterial angiograms of electrically injured extremities, no vascular changes could be found. The observed changes may more likely be explained by vascular changes similar to ischemia-reperfusion injury with immediate cessation of capillary blood flow in response to current passage. This event seems to be followed by vascular spasms lasting for an extended time, with subsequent vasodilation and restoration of flow.[47–49]

Physical therapy and functional splinting is ongoing and is begun on the day of admission. The "anti-claw" position is utilized in hand injuries to prevent contractures. Custom splints are fabricated on the unit by Occupational Therapy personnel. In addition, active and passive range of motion is instituted along with elevation of the extremity to decrease the risk of edema-related complications. The need for surgical fixation is greatly reduced with an early aggressive approach to splinting. In the authors' institution arthrodesis is a last resort, occurring only once or twice per year,

providing yet another reason for early referral to the burn center. Early active participation of the Physical Medicine and Rehabilitation department is essential to improved functional outcomes. In most burn centers a weekly or biweekly multidisciplinary conference is held to discuss all patient needs, both in the acute and outpatient settings.

Serial neuromuscular examinations are performed to document neurologic status. Neurologic deficits may present on admission or develop over days to weeks, with late-onset neurologic complications occurring up to 2 years post injury. Regional anesthesia is therefore avoided to minimize medicolegal issues should a late-onset deficit occur after surgical procedures.

DIAGNOSTIC ADJUNCTS

Multiple diagnostic modalities have been investigated; attempting to accelerate the process of identifying the extent of deep tissue necrosis. Radionuclide scanning with xenon-133[50] and technetium pyrophosphate[51,52] have been shown to be accurate predictors of tissue damage. Hammond showed that scanning did not, however, decrease hospital stay or number of operations required.[52] Magnetic resonance imaging (MRI) provides poor sensitivity for evaluation of muscle damage in nonperfused areas. Gadolinium-enhanced MRI demonstrates potential viability in zones of tissue edema.[1,53,54] In general, however, these diagnostic scans add little to direct clinical evaluation and are not currently employed in most centers. The authors have used them in select instances such as difficult cases wherein a patient is in denial about the need for amputation. The scans can be used as added evidence in the doctor-patient discussion regarding timing and need for these disfiguring amputations.

DIFFICULT WOUNDS

Contact points to areas such as the scalp, chest, and abdomen require special attention and expertise. Scalp burns require extra considerations. First, contact points buried within thick scalp hair may be missed if the examiner does not search for them, then to become issues later. Scalp contact points also imply a transfer of electric current through the CNS. This event should alert the team to possible complications such as brain and spinal cord injury that can be seen in the absence of trauma. The clinician should maintain a low threshold for obtaining computed tomography scans of the head and spine in these cases; given that neurologic complications secondary to electrical injury often present in a delayed fashion.

Timely diagnosis can have medicolegal implications in this setting. Scalp burns that spare the galea are relatively straightforward in that simple excision and grafting is routinely successful. Wounds that penetrate to bone, however, require a different approach. In areas that penetrate into the outer table a viable wound bed can be provided by removing dead bone with an osteotome or a high-speed orthopedic drill with burr attachment. Care must be exercised to avoid penetrating to dura or deeper structures. If dura is exposed and the area is small, these wounds can be expected to granulate without causing CNS infection, providing the area can be kept from desiccating and hence opening. This process usually requires multiple trips to the operating room, conservative serial debridement, and weeks to months of meticulous wound care. Silver sulfadiazine dressings may be used initially on the exposed bone, which is helpful in preventing wound desiccation, followed by Sulfamylon solution once granulation tissue forms. The best and most expedient approach to these deep skull wounds, however, is a rotational scalp flap over the burned area. Split-thickness skin grafts cover the resulting adjacent defect. This procedure provides rapid closure and minimal morbidity. Skin expansion of the hair-bearing area can be performed 12 to 18 months later to obliterate the areas of alopecia. Large and complex scalp wounds, in particular those including facial structures, will require free tissue transfer, utilizing recipient vessels outside the zone of injury, usually in the neck. This procedure requires a multi-team approach, with the plastic surgery team and in some cases the neurosurgeons. It is good policy to consult these services early in the patient's course when one expects a need for their expertise.

Complex chest wall injuries present additional closure problems. These may include exposed bone and cartilage in locations adjacent to or remote from soft tissue flaps. The role of the burn surgeon is to remove nonviable tissue and obtain coverage. A sign of maturity in the burn surgeon is the realization that one cannot fix everything. With this in mind, a simple approach is usually most beneficial to the patient and when this is not possible consultation with specialty services again is in order. Costal chondritis is the most frequent complication of deep chest wall burns, which can be a source of long-term morbidity, requiring multiple operative debridements.

Abdominal wounds provide the potential for internal injuries both directly under the contact points and remotely as a result of late ischemic necrosis.[55,56] Diagnosis of these injuries is problematic. Patients with larger significant injuries often present a complex diagnostic problem. These patients are often receiving large doses of narcotic analgesics, and have bulky dressings in place and a significant inflammatory response, thus adding to diagnostic uncertainty. General deterioration, in particular feeding intolerance, should prompt laparotomy to rule out intra-abdominal complication. Large abdominal defects require careful planning and often input from specialty surgical services.

Low-voltage burns of the oral cavity are the most common type of serious electrical burn in young children.[57] Most of these injuries are the result of an unattended small child (commonly <4 years of age) chewing on an electric cord. The more common isolated commissure injuries are managed on an outpatient basis providing there are no general burn or social issues requiring inpatient management. If the eschar separates there is a risk of labial artery bleeding that has been reported to occur between 1 to 2 weeks post burn. Precautions to parents should include instructions to apply direct pressure and return immediately to the emergency department should this occur.[58] Although this complication is reported in every published article on the topic, the senior author has yet to come across such a complication after almost 30 years of practice. Early surgical debridement is usually not recommended for the commissure burn. Burns of the center portion of the lip may require early aggressive debridement and closure. Local wound care consists of cleaning the wound with hydrogen peroxide and application of an antibacterial agent such as bacitracin. Following healing, treatment varies by severity of injury. Gentle stretching and the use of oral splinting gives a good cosmetic and functional result in most patients, with reconstructive surgery being reserved for the remainder. A mucosal advancement flap may be used for severe microstomia.

LIGHTNING INJURY

Virtually all lightning injuries and death can be prevented by taking appropriate precautions.[59] Approximately 100,000 thunderstorms occur in the United States each year with lightning killing more people than other weather phenomena. Lightning causes approximately 80 fatalities per year, with Florida and Texas having the most deaths.[60–63] Lightning involves a single massive current impulse that is roughly equivalent to a direct current strike of 2000 to 2 billion volts of extremely short duration (0.1–1 milliseconds). Electrocution by lightning is not a reportable injury, and accurate statistics are lacking. Lightning may cause full cardiac arrest by inducing asystole or central apnea. Although massive cardiac depolarization leads to asystole, the heart's automaticity usually restarts the heart in normal sinus rhythm. Depolarization of the brain is believed to stun the respiratory center, causing central apnea.[59] Prompt cardiopulmonary resuscitation is especially effective in these injuries.[64] Major cutaneous injury is rare unless a nearby object is turned incandescent, causing a flash/flame type injury. In a recent large series published from the authors' institution mean cutaneous burn size was just under 7% TBSA in lightning-injured patients. The pathognomonic cutaneous sign of lightning strike is a dendritic, fernlike, branching erythematous pattern on the skin (Lichtenberg figure), which appears within an hour of injury and fades rapidly. Full-thickness injury is not common with the exception of burns on the tips of the toes reportedly being somewhat characteristic.[65] Another common finding is tympanic membrane rupture, along with injuries to the middle and inner ear.[66] The frequency of these injuries thus mandates good otoscopic examination. There is, however, no need for initial consultation from ear/nose/throat specialists unless injury is present.

Neurologic complications include loss of consciousness, seizures, paresthesias, and paralysis, which may develop over several days post injury. Lightning paralysis or keraunoparalysis is a term used to describe the rare transient paralysis associated with the extreme vasoconstriction and sensory disturbances of one or more extremities seen in this patient population. This paralysis typically resolves within hours but may last up to a full day.[67] Surgically treatable lesions must be ruled out; these include epidural, subdural, and intracerebral hematomas. Altered levels of consciousness should alert the clinician to this possibility and prompt an immediate computed tomography scan.[62] The prognosis of many lightning-caused neurologic injuries is generally better than for other types of traumatic brain injury. A recent report of 10 patients with follow-up 12 years post injury showed that none had long-term neurologic or psychological deficits.[68]

COMPLICATIONS

Early complications consist of renal, septic, cardiac, neurologic, and ocular manifestations. Renal dysfunction in high-voltage electrical injury occurs in approximately 10% of patients secondary to hypovolemia- or rhabdomyolysis-induced acute tubular necrosis. This complication should be easily avoided by the vigilant clinician.

Cardiac damage is recognized and treated on admission. As discussed earlier, late-occurring arrhythmias are rare. Myocardial infarction is rare, but has been reported in a small number of patients.

Cataract formation is the most common ocular complication of electrical injuries.[69,70] The incidence of premature cataract formation has been reported to occur in as many as 5% to 20% of patients after electrical injury.[71,72] Surprisingly, cataracts occur equally in patients who have obvious contact points on the face or head and in those who do not. In addition, there is a high degree of bilaterality in these injuries. Approximately 70% of these cataracts eventually progress to the point of requiring surgery, the results of which are uniformly good. The latent period may range from weeks to years, with the mean being 6 months.[71] Ophthalmologic examination in these patients can therefore be helpful for purposes of workmen's compensation claims, to document visual acuity before complications in the event one occurs in the future. This examination helps sort injury-related complication from preexisting problems.

Neurologic complications are common sequelae of high-voltage electrical injuries and can affect the brain, spinal cord, and peripheral nerves. Immediate but frequently transient symptoms include varying levels of unconsciousness, respiratory paralysis, and motor paralysis. Permanent changes include cortical encephalopathy, caused by the electric injury itself or resulting from hypoxia at the time of injury.[73] Spinal cord injuries are rare but may present as progressive muscular atrophy, amyotrophic lateral sclerosis, or transverse myelitis. This diverse set of complications may present early or late (in the first days or up to 2 years after injury), mandating a thorough neurologic examination on admission and before discharge. A study of 90 patients with electrical injuries was conducted at the University of Washington Burn Center to identify and evaluate neurologic complications.[9] There were four deaths. Of the remainder, 11 of 22 low-voltage injured patients had immediate neurologic symptoms; 9 of whom had resolution of symptoms. Of the 64 patients with high-voltage injuries, 67% developed immediate central or peripheral neurologic symptoms. One-third had peripheral neuropathies with one-third of those persistent. Twelve percent had delayed-onset peripheral neuropathy with 50% of those resolving. No late-onset central neuropathies were reported. Spinal cord injury caused by high-voltage electricity may be the result of trauma or a delayed-onset neurologic complication related to the passage of current through the nervous system. The reported incidence of spinal cord injury after high-voltage electric trauma ranges between 2% and 27%. Mechanical damage of the spinal cord is an important consideration, because victims often sustain a fall from a height after high-voltage injuries. Spinal cord compression may also result from tetanic muscle contraction of the paraspinous muscles during electrical shock. The estimated incidence of delayed electrical spinal cord injury has been reported to range from less than 1% to 6%.[74–77] Ko reported on 13 patients with delayed-onset spinal cord injuries, postulating on a vascular cause of the deficit.[78] In general, resolution of early-onset lesions is much better than for late onset, spasticity is more common than flaccidity, and function is affected more than sensation. Sympathetic overactivity with changes in bowel habits, and urinary and sexual function is the primary autonomic complex complication. Although the exact mechanism of nerve injury has not been explained, direct injury by electrical current and vascular causes have received the most attention. To date, imaging studies, including angiography and MRI, have not been helpful in predicting or evaluating the extent of deficit. Somatosensory-evoked potentials may be useful in the diagnosis and long-term follow-up of these patients. Early involvement of an experienced, interested physiatrist is important in assessing long-term needs and developing a therapy plan. Early rehabilitation is therefore essential and another of the services available in the modern verified burn center.

Posttraumatic stress disorder is more common after electrical burns than after thermal burns. General rehabilitation and self-assessed quality of life are, however, comparable after thermal burns and electrical burns.[79,80] In a study comparing electrical burn patients with nonburned electricians, Pliskin showed significantly higher cognitive, physical, and emotional complaints not related to injury or litigation status in the injured individuals.[81]

Heterotopic ossification (HO) occurring at the cut ends of amputation sites is unique to electrically burned patients. HO will occur in about 80% of patients with long bone amputations, but not in patients with disarticulations or small bone amputations. Surgical intervention in these patients has been reported in 28% of these cases.[82] Patients with large TBSA cutaneous thermal injuries have heterotopic calcification in periarticular tissue of large joints, most commonly the elbows. Causative factors include forced passive mobilization, secondary articular bleeding, and calcium precipitation and deposition in damaged or degenerating muscle and connective tissue.

Electrical injuries make up a relatively small proportion of total burn unit admissions. These injuries, however, consume enormous resources in both direct and indirect cost to society. Much of this cost is difficult to calculate and represents lost wages and long-term disability in young, previously working individuals. This situation is related to the fact that most of these injuries occur in younger adults while performing work-related activities.[4,83–85] These injuries can be expected to remain costly to the individual and our society at large. As a result careful planning, a team approach with good communication is required for optimal care.

REFERENCES

1. Lee RC. Injury by electrical forces: pathophysiology, manifestations and therapy. Curr Probl Surg 1997; 34:738–40.
2. Esselman PC, Thombs BD, Magyar-Russell G, et al. Burn rehabilitation: state of the science. Am J Phys Med Rehabil 2006;85:383–418.
3. Purdue GF, Arnoldo BD, Hunt JL. Electric injuries. In: Herndon DN, editor. Total burn care: text and atlas. 3rd edition. Philadelphia: Elsevier; 2007. p. 513–20.
4. Arnoldo BD, Purdue GF, Kowalske K, et al. Electrical Injuries: a 20-year review. J Burn Care Rehabil 2004; 25:479–84.
5. Janicak CA. Occupational fatalities caused by contact with overhead power lines in the construction industry. J Occup Environ Med 1997;39:328–32.
6. Merriam-Webster Online Dictionary, 2008.
7. Hunt JL, Mason AD, Masterson TS, et al. The pathophysiology of acute electric injuries. J Trauma 1976; 16:335–40.
8. Jain S, Bandi V. Electrical and lightning injuries. Crit Care Clin 1999;15:319–31.
9. Grube BJ, Heimbach DM, Engrav LH, et al. Neurologic consequences of electrical burns. J Trauma 1990;30:254–8.
10. Hunt JL, McManus WF, Haney WP, et al. Vascular lesions in acute electric injuries. J Trauma 1974;14: 461–73.
11. Nichter LS, Bryant CA, Kenney JG, et al. Injuries due to commercial electric current. J Burn Care Rehabil 1984;5:124–37.
12. Tuttnauer A, Mordzynski SC, Weiss YG. Electrical and lightning injuries. Contemp Crit Care 2006;7:1–10.
13. Lee RC, Zhang D, Hannig J. Biophysical injury mechanisms in electrical shock trauma. Annu Rev Biomed Eng 2000;2:477–509.
14. Block TA, Aarsvold JN, Matthews KL, et al. The 1995 Lindberg Award. Nonthermally mediated muscle injury and necrosis in electrical trauma. J Burn Care Rehabil 1995;16:581–8.

15. DeBono R. A histological analysis of a high voltage electric current injury to an upper limb. Burns 1999;25:541–7.

16. Chen W, Lee RC. Altered ion channel conductance and ionic selectivity induced by large imposed membrane potential pulse. Biophys J 1994;67:603–12.

17. Layton TR, McMurty JM, McClain EJ, et al. Multiple spine fractures from electric injury. J Burn Care Rehabil 1984;5:373–5.

18. Baxter CR, Shires T. Physiological response to crystalloid resuscitation of severe burns. Ann N Y Acad Sci 1968;150:874–94.

19. Yiannis SC, Gesthimani M, Apostolos I, et al. The syndrome of rhabdomyolysis: complications and treatment. Eur J Intern Med 2008;19:568–74.

20. Heyman SN, Rosen S, Fuchs S, et al. Myoglobinuric acute renal failure in rat: a role for medullary hypoperfusion, hypoxia and tubular obstruction. J Am Soc Nephrol 1996;7:1066–74.

21. Thadhani R, Pascual M, Bonventre JV. Acute renal failure. N Engl J Med 1996;334:1448–60.

22. Zager RA, Gamelin LM. Pathogenic mechanisms in experimental hemoglobinuric acute renal failure. Am J Physiol 1989;256(3Pt 2):F446–55.

23. Yowler CJ, Fratianne RB. Current status of burn resuscitation. Clin Plast Surg 2000;27(1):1–10.

24. Pham TM, Gibran NS. Thermal and electrical injuries. Surg Clin North Am 2007;87:185–206.

25. Holt SG, Moore KP. Pathogenesis and treatment of renal dysfunction in rhabdomyolysis. Intensive Care Med 2001;27:803–11.

26. Brown CV, Rhee P, Chan L, et al. Preventing renal failure in patients with rhabdomyolysis: do bicarbonate and mannitol make a difference? J Trauma 2004;56:1191–6.

27. Arnoldo BD, Klein M, Gibran NS. Practice guidelines for the management of electrical injuries. J Burn Care Res 2006;27(4):439–47.

28. Bailey B, Gaudreault P, Thiviege RL. Experience with guidelines for cardiac monitoring after electric injury in children. Am J Emerg Med 2000;18:671–5.

29. Hunt JL, Sato RM, Baxter CR. Acute electric burns. Arch Surg 1980;115:434–8.

30. Purdue GF, Hunt JL. Electrocardiographic monitoring after electrical injury: necessity or luxury. J Trauma 1986;26:166–7.

31. Housinger TA, Green L, Shahanigan S, et al. A prospective study of myocardial damage in electrical injuries. J Trauma 1985;25:122–4.

32. McBride JW, Labrosse KR, McCoy HG, et al. Is serum creatine kinase-MB in electrically injured patients predictive of myocardial injury? JAMA 1986;255:764–8.

33. Dilworth D, Hasan D, Alford P, et al. Evaluation of myocardial injury in electrical burn patients [abstract]. J Burn Care Rehabil 1998;19(Pt 2): S239.

34. Luce E, Gottlieb SE. "True" high-tension electrical injuries. Ann Plast Surg 1984;12:321–6.

35. Achauer B, Applebaum R, Vander Kam VM. Electric burn injury to the upper extremity. Br J Plast Surg 1994;47:331–40.

36. Mann RJ, Wallquist JM. Early fasciotomy in the treatment of high-voltage electrical burns of the extremities. South Med J 1975;68:1103–8.

37. D'Amato TA, Kaplan JB, Britt LD. High-voltage electrical injury: a role for mandatory exploration of deep muscle compartments. J Natl Med Assoc 1994;86: 535–7.

38. Mann R, Gibran N, Engrav L, et al. Is immediate decompression of high voltage electrical injuries to the upper extremity always necessary. J Trauma 1996;40(4):584–9.

39. Koop J, Loos B, Spilker G, et al. Correlation between serum creatinine kinase levels and extent of muscle damage in electrical burns. Burns 2004; 30:680–3.

40. Moylan J, Wellford W, Pruitt B. Circulator changes following circumferential extremity burns evaluated by ultrasonic flowmeter: an analysis of 60 thermally injured limbs. J Trauma 1971;11:763–849.

41. Salisbury R, McKeel D, Mason A. Ischemic necrosis of intrinsic muscles of the hand after thermal injuries. J Bone Joint Surg 1974;56A:1701–7.

42. Botte MJ, Gelberman RH. Acute compartment syndrome of the forearm. Hand Clin 1998;14(3): 391–403.

43. Gelberman RH. Volkmann's contracture of the upper extremity: pathophysiology and reconstruction. In: Mubarak SJ, Hargens AR, editors, Compartment syndrome and Volkmann's contracture (Monographs in clinical orthopaedics), vol. 3. Philadelphia: WB Saunders; 1981.

44. Gelberman RH, Garfin SR, Hergenroeder PT, et al. Compartment syndrome of the forearm: diagnosis and treatment. Clin Orthop 1981;161:252–61.

45. Gelberman RH, Zakaib GS, Mubarak SJ, et al. Decompression of forearm compartment syndromes. Clin Orthop 1978;134:225–9.

46. Berman SS, Schilling JD, McIntyre KE, et al. Shoelace technique for delayed primary closure of fasciotomies. Am J Surg 1994;167:435–6.

47. Vogt PM, Niederbichler AD, Spies M, et al. Electric injury: reconstructive problems. In: Herndon DN, editor. Total burn care: text and atlas. 3rd edition. Philadelphia: Elsevier; 2007. p. 521–9.

48. Hussman J, Zamboni WA, Russel RC, et al. A model for recording the microcirculatory changes associated with standardized electrical injury of skeletal muscle. J Surg Res 1995;59:725–32.

49. Ponten B, Erikson U, Johansson SH, et al. New observations on tissue changes along the pathway of the current in an electrical injury. Scand J Plast Reconstr Surg 1970;4:75–82.

50. Clayton JM, Hayes AC, Hammond J, et al. Xenon-133 determination of muscle blood flow in electrical injury. J Trauma 1977;17:293–8.

51. Hunt JL, Lewis S, Parkey R, et al. The use of technetium 99 stannous pyrophosphate scintigraphy to identify muscle damage in acute electric burns. J Trauma 1979;19:409–13.

52. Hammond J, Ward CG. The use of technetium-99 pyrophosphate scanning in management of high voltage electrical injuries. Am Surg 1994;68:886–8.

53. Fleckenstein JL, Chasson DP, Bonte FJ, et al. High-voltage electric injury: assessment of muscle viability with MR imaging and Tc-99 pyrophosphate scintigraphy. Radiology 1993;195:205–10.

54. Ohashi M, Koizumi J, Hosoda Y, et al. Correlation between magnetic resonance imaging and histopathology of an amputated forearm after electric injury. Burns 1998;24:362–8.

55. Newsome TW, Curreri PW, Kurenius K. Visceral injuries—an unusual complication of an electrical burn. Arch Surg 1972;105:494–7.

56. Reilley AF, Rees R, Kelton P, et al. Abdominal aortic occlusion following electric injury. J Burn Care Rehabil 1985;6:226–9.

57. Rai J, Jeschke MG, Barrow RE, et al. Electrical injuries: a 30-year review. J Trauma 1999;46:933–6.

58. Orgel MG, Brown HC, Woolhouse FM. Electrical burns in the mouth of children: a method for assessing results. J Trauma 1975;15:285–9.

59. Maghsoudi H, Adyani Y, Ahmadian N. Electric and lightning injuries. J Burn Care Res 2007;28:255–61.

60. Centers for Disease Control. Lightning associated death—United States 1980–1995. Morb Mortal Wkly Rep 1998;47:391–4.

61. Lopez RE, Holle RL. Demographics of lightning casualties. Semin Neurol 1995;15:286–95.

62. Hiestand D, Colice GL. Lightning-strike injury. J Intensive Care Med 1988;3:303–14.

63. Trible CG, Persing JA, Morgan RF, et al. Lightning injury. Curr Concept Trauma Care 1984;5–10.

64. Moran KT, Thupari JN, Munster AM. Electric and lightning induced cardiac arrest reversed by prompt cardiopulmonary resuscitation. JAMA 1986;255:2157–61.

65. Fahmy FS, Brinsden MD, Smith J, et al. Lightning: the multisystem group injuries. J Trauma 1999;46:937–40.

66. Bergstrom L, Neblett LM, Sando I, et al. The lightning damaged ear. Arch Otolaryngol 1974;100:117–21.

67. Duis HJ, Klasen HJ, Reenalda P. Keraunoparalysis, a 'specific' lightning injury. Burns Incl Therm Inj 1985;12:54–7.

68. Muehlberger T, Vogt PM, Munster AM. The long-term consequences of lightning injuries. Burns 2001;27:829–33.

69. Johnson EV, Klein LB, Skalka HW. Electrical cataracts: a case report and review of literature. Ophthalmic Surg 1987;18:283–5.

70. Boozalis GT, Purdue GF, Hunt JP, et al. Ocular changes from electrical burn injuries: a literature review and report of cases. J Burn Care Rehabil 1991;5:458–62.

71. Saffle JR, Crandall A, Warden GD. Cataracts: a long term complication of electrical injury. J Trauma 1985;25:17–21.

72. Reddy SC. Electrical cataracts: a case report and review of the literature. Eur J Ophthalmol 1999;9:134–8.

73. Heimbach DM, Gibran NS. Miscellaneous burns and cold injuries. In: Souba WW, Fink MP, Jurkovich GJ, et al, editors. ACS surgery principles & practice. 6th edition; BC Decker. p. 1437–48.

74. Arevalo JM, Lorente JA, Balseiro-Gomez J. Spinal cord injury after electrical trauma treated in a burn unit. Burns 1999;25:449–52.

75. Varghese G, Mani MM, Redford JB. Spinal cord injuries following electrical accidents. Paraplegia 1986;24:309–14.

76. Koller J, Orsagh J. Delayed neurological sequelae of high-tension electrical burn. Burns 1989;15:175–8.

77. Winkelman MD. Neurological complications of thermal and electrical burns. In: Aminoff MJ, editor. Neurology and general medicine. New York: Churchill Livingstone; 1995. p. 915–29.

78. Ko SH, Chun W, Kim HC. Delayed spinal cord injury following electrical burns: A 7-year experience. Burns 2004;30:691–5.

79. Mancusi-Ungaro HR Jr, Tarbox AR, Wainwright DJ. Posttraumatic stress disorder in electric burn patients. J Burn Care Rehabil 1986;7:521–5.

80. Cochran A, Edelman LS, Saffle JR, et al. Self-reported quality of life after electrical and thermal injury. J Burn Care Rehabil 2004;25:61–6.

81. Pliskin NH, Capelli-Schellpfeffer M, Law RT, et al. Neuropsychological symptom presentation after electrical injury. J Trauma 1998;44:709–15.

82. Helm PA, Walker SC. New bone formation in electrically burn-injured patients. Arch Phys Med Rehabil 1987;68:284–6.

83. Butler ED, Grant TD. Electrical injuries, with specific reference to the upper extremities: a review of 182 cases. Am J Surg 1977;134:95–101.

84. Skoog T. Electrical injuries. J Trauma 1970;10:816–30.

85. Wilkinson C, Wood M. High voltage electric injury. Am J Surg 1978;136:693–6.

Cold Injury

Wm J. Mohr, MD[a,b,*], Kamrun Jenabzadeh, MD[c],
David H. Ahrenholz, MD[a,b]

KEYWORDS

- Frostbite • Cold injury • Intra-arterial thrombolytic therapy
- Amputation • Angiogram

HISTORICAL IMPACT OF COLD

Man is a warm-blooded organism best suited to a tropical environment with temperatures around 81°F (27°C).[1] Our sense of adventure and entitlement has led us to live in climates not ideally suited to our existence. Although we have some ability to adapt to colder climes, most of our survival is due to behavioral changes in response to the weather conditions. When we impair our ability to prepare adequately for freezing temperatures, we place ourselves at risk for cold injuries.

Throughout history man has paid a price for living in cold climates. The oldest documented case of frostbite was recognized in a mummy found in the Chilean mountains, and dates back 5000 years.[2] Hippocrates recognized that tissues with frostbite blistered after warming,[3] Celsus provided the first description of tissue necrosis with frostbite,[4] and Baron Dominique Larrey, Napoleon's military surgeon, gave the first description of the devastation of freeze-thaw-freeze injury in French troops retreating from Moscow.[5] Subsequent study has clarified the physiology and laid the groundwork for our current treatment of frostbite.

It is clear that military and world history has been changed several times by cold weather. Xenophon lost half of his 10,000-man Spartan army in the Carduchian Mountains of Armenia in 400 BC.[6,7] The armies of Charles XII of Sweden, the Napoleon, and Hitler all fell victim to the Russian winter.[8–10]

The German army sustained 250,000 cases of frostbite in the attack on Moscow and resulted in 20,000 amputations in the winter of 1941 to 1942.[6,7] Combined troops lost to cold injuries in World War I were more than 280,000.[7] Although military personnel still risk cold injury in harsh weather conditions, frostbite today is a disease predominantly of civilian populations, particularly among the indigent, intoxicated, and the mentally ill.

EPIDEMIOLOGY/PREDISPOSITION

Many factors increase the risk of cold injury. The majority of civilian frostbite injuries are associated with mental impairment related to mental illness (10%–100%),[11,12] alcohol consumption (35%–53%),[11,13–15] or drug use (4%).[14,16] Alcohol and sedative drugs decrease the awareness of cold and impair the judgment necessary to seek shelter.[17] Alcohol also inhibits shivering and causes cutaneous vasodilatation,[18] precipitating frostbite at warmer temperatures (−8°F [−22°C] vs −20°F [−30°C]).[15] Many schizophrenic patients exhibit acrocyanosis,[19] and their ability to assess tissue cooling or comprehend cold injury is often impaired. Any behavior that prolongs the cold exposure will worsen the prognosis.[20] There are several known risk factors associated with the development of frostbite (**Box 1**). Identification of the causative factors is important for prevention of recurrent cold injuries. A growing participation in winter sports and outdoor activities,[9,21,22]

Disclosure: None of the authors has a financial interest in any of the products, devices, or drugs mentioned in the article.

[a] The Burn Center, Department of Trauma and General Surgery, Regions Hospital, Mail Stop 11105C, 640 Jackson Street, St. Paul, MN 55101, USA

[b] Department of Surgery, University of Minnesota, Mail Stop 11105C, 640 Jackson Street, St. Paul, MN 55101, USA

[c] University of Minnesota, Mail Stop 11105C, 640 Jackson Street, St. Paul, MN 55101, USA

* Corresponding author. The Burn Center, Division of Trauma, Burn and Critical Care, Regions Hospital, Mail Stop 11105C, 640 Jackson Street, St. Paul, MN 55101.
E-mail address: william.j.mohr@healthpartners.com (W. J. Mohr).

Hand Clin 25 (2009) 481–496
doi:10.1016/j.hcl.2009.06.004

hand.theclinics.com

Box 1
Risk factors for frostbite

The intoxicated (alcohol, other drugs)

The incompetent (mental illness or dementia)

The infirm (elderly, especially with falls)

The insensate (diabetes, neuropathy, paraplegia)

The inexperienced (new to cold climates)

The inducted (wartime increases risk)

The indigent (homeless)

---

combined with persons who become stranded while traveling, now account for up to one-third of cold injuries.[11,14] The extremities are the most susceptible sites; hands and feet account for 90% of reported injuries.[20] Preparation for emergencies is the key for survival and to avoid injuries. In Minnesota, local media remind residents yearly to prepare a car emergency kit as winter approaches.

Although under identical conditions, infants and the elderly are more susceptible to local cold injuries,[23] they are not prone to the behaviors that promote cold exposure. Adult men, aged 30 to 49 years, are the most commonly affected.[14,24] Because muscle and fat have insulation properties, body mass may be more important than age or body surface area.[25] Malnutrition and exertion decrease the fuel available for heat generation.[25] Many medical problems may contribute to the extent of the cold injuries, but are rarely the sole cause in our experience.

The authors have reviewed the predisposing factors in 133 patients with severe frostbite admitted to the regional burn center over a 17-year period. Approximately 80% were men and their mean age was 40 years. The authors found 50% of these patients had documented alcoholism or an elevated blood alcohol level, 24% were positive for drugs of abuse, 59% were smokers, 29% had major mental health diagnoses, and 20% were homeless. Almost 30% had greater than a 24-hour delay to definitive treatment, either due to poor decisions following the injury or because of weather related issues. Hands were frequently affected (48%), with 26% of patients having only hand frostbite.[26]

In the absence of wind, skin can freeze at 28°F (−2°C). Freeze injury to exposed skin occurs in 1 hour with a temperature of 0°F (−18°C) and a 10 mph wind, but in 30 minutes with a 20 mph wind. The wind speed accelerates the heat loss by convection, defined as the wind chill temperature.[27]

As the wind chill reaches approximately −40°F (−40°C), tissue freezing occurs in minutes. Although tissue freezes more quickly at lower temperatures, the degree of irreversible damage is related to the length of time the tissue remains frozen, not the final temperature of the injured tissue.[27]

SPECTRUM OF INJURY

Frostbite is the most common local cold injury, although not all cold exposure results in tissue freezing.[28] There is a continuum that ranges from minimal skin chilling to frank tissue crystallization from exposure to subfreezing temperatures.[29,30] There are two key factors that categorize these injuries, the rate of cooling and the ultimate presence or absence of ice crystals in the tissues (**Box 1**). A patient may have a combination of these injuries in different body parts following a cold exposure.

Frostnip represents a mild cold injury and is completely reversible. This injury is characterized by skin pallor and numbness,[9,31] and the rapid temperature drop causes local pain.[29] It is seen typically on the face and hands. There is no ice crystal formation and no tissue damage. The warmed tissue becomes hyperemic without blistering, and decreased sensation or tingling may persist for weeks.[29,31]

Chilblain (pernio) results from repeated exposure to near freezing temperatures and is a more severe form of cold injury, but has no ice crystal formation.[29,31] A chronic vasculitis develops and is usually located on the face, anterior lower leg, the hands, and feet.[29,31] The skin has a violaceous color with plaques or nodules, and patients exhibit pain and pruritus with cold exposure.[29] The calcium channel blocker nifedipine significantly reduces the pain and time to healing of this condition, although many cases are self-limited.[29,32]

Frostbite occurs when tissues freeze slowly and form ice crystals. The temperatures necessary to produce this injury are typically less than 28°F (−2°C). The injuries are circumferential, progress distal to proximal, and are potentially reversible.

Flash freeze injury causes extremely rapid cooling and formation of intracellular ice crystals. The mechanism is contact with cold metals or volatile liquids. These injuries have a rapid onset, occur along a body surface plane and are almost never circumferential.

PATHOPHYSIOLOGY

The body's thermostat for temperature regulation is the hypothalamus with sensors located in the skin and core.[33] This system allows us to maintain tight control of our temperature, varying from 101.3°F (38.5°C) in the liver, 100.4°F (38°C) in the rectum, 98.6°F (37°C) under the tongue, and 89.6°F (32°C) in the skin at room temperature.[8] At rest and under most conditions, the body can produce more heat than it needs. When in a positive heat balance, the skin temperature of the digits is higher than the more proximal parts.[34] In fact, the skin has the ability to alter blood flow by a factor of 200.[35] As environmental temperatures drop, the body responds by increasing heat production and limiting skin blood flow to prevent further heat loss. This system serves to preserve life but at the potential expense of the limbs, leading to a constellation of problems referred to as local cold injuries, based on the rate of cooling and the formation of ice crystals in the tissue (**Table 1**).

The blood flow to the skin is one of the most important means of heat regulation.[31] The extremities account for 50% of the body surface area[9] but are responsible for most of the protective response to the cold, because the skin covering the head and trunk have little capacity for vasoconstriction.[33] The skin contains 3 to 10 times more receptors for cold than for heat.[36] In response to cold exposure, the body tries to preserve temperature (vasoconstriction) and attempts to generate more heat energy (shivering).

Shivering is an involuntary response to the cold. It begins when the core temperature falls below 98.6 (37°C) or the skin temperature drops below 80.6°F (27°C).[33,37] Shivering is the result of disorganized contractions in opposing muscle groups at a rate of 6 to 12 cycles/s, as blood from the core is shunted to the muscles and the skin surface. This procedure can generate about 500 kcal/h, but is extremely inefficient and nonproductive work. Heat losses are increased by about 25% in this fashion and may double or triple the oxygen consumption.[33]

The "hunting reflex" describes alternating cycles of vasoconstriction and vasodilation in the peripheral circulation mediated by the sympathetic nervous system.[38] Initial vasoconstriction reduces the blood flow to the skin and subcutaneous tissues by 10-fold,[33] and increases the

Table 1		
Classification of local cold injury		
Cooling	**No Tissue Ice**	**Tissue Ice**
Rapid	Frostnip	Flash freeze injury
Slow	Chilblains or pernio	Frostbite

Data from Ahrenholz DH. Frostbite. Problems Gen Surg 2003;20(1):130.

thermal insulation of superficial tissues by more than 300%.[37] These combined effects can produce an initial increase in the core temperature of about 0.9°F (0.5°C).[33] Although the blood flow is diverted away from the skin, the tissues are hypoxic and subject to rapid freezing. The blood vessels dilate every 5 to 10 minutes providing a bolus of heat and oxygen to the affected extremity, which adversely affects the core temperature. When the temperature approaches 82°F (28°C), the reflex is lost and vasoconstriction persists until rewarming occurs.[4] At this temperature, even the shivering mechanism fails, leaving the body essentially poikilothermic and unable to protect itself from further cold stress.[33]

Tissue Freezing

Local tissue damage is influenced by the susceptibility of specific body tissues to cold, the rate of cooling, the lowest tissue temperature achieved, the duration of the cold exposure, duration of ischemia, and the rewarming conditions.[4,28,29] Although the skin freezes sooner at lower temperatures, tissue destruction is more dependent on the total time the tissue is frozen.[10,28] There are two mechanisms of cellular damage: tissue freezing and reperfusion injury.[9,20,28,31] The latter is more critical, due to thrombosis and progressive cellular hypoxia resulting in a time dependent cell death phenomenon.[10,29,30]

Shivering stops at a core temperature of approximately 82°F (28°C); skin temperatures then approach the ambient temperature until 28°F (−2°C), when ice crystals slowly form in the extracellular fluid (**Fig. 1**). This reaction releases considerable heat (79 cal/g), and the tissue temperature plateaus.[1] Under conditions of slow cooling, the extracellular ice crystals gradually increase in size and the concentrated solutes draw water out of the adjacent cells. The deflating cells become less subject to puncture by the growing ice spicules.[29,31] Cellular dehydration alters the protein and lipid composition of the cell membranes rendering them less stable. The cellular pH falls and disrupts the physiologic activity.[39,40]

As freezing progresses, ice crystals form in the plasma causing vascular sludging.[9] Blood viscosity rises, cells aggregate and occlude capillaries and other small vessels.[41] Cells that survive dehydration and mechanical disruption from ice crystals are exposed to a 10-fold increase in the cellular sodium concentration, which can denature the cell membranes.[10] Despite these processes, cell death is not inevitable due to the decreased metabolic activity of the frozen tissue. Nerve, cartilage, bone, and especially the endothelial cells are

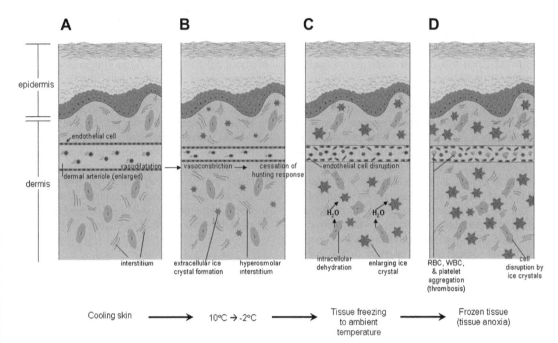

Fig. 1. Tissue freezing. (*A*) Skin is exposed to cool environment. (*B*) As temperature declines, the hunting response ceases. Early ice crystal formation begins. (*C*) Freezing disrupts endothelial cell integrity. Water exits cells to contribute to growing extracellular ice crystals. (*D*) Circulatory stasis secondary to thrombosis and cell sludging results in tissue anoxia. RBC, red blood cell; WBC, white blood cell. (*Adapted from* Britt LD, Dascombe WH, Rodriguez A. New horizons in management of hypothermia and frostbite injury. Surg Clin North Am 1991;71(2):360; with permission.)

damaged more quickly than are skin, fat, or connective tissue.[4,9,42] As the tissue temperature falls below −4°F (−20°C), 90% of the tissue water of the limb is frozen.[43] From that point, the tissue temperature falls rapidly to the surrounding temperature.[4]

True frostbite injuries are caused by a slow cooling process.[9,29] When freezing occurs rapidly, defined as greater than 10°C per minute drop in tissue temperature, intracellular and extracellular ice crystals form and lyse the cells.[44–46] Flash freeze injuries occur following contact with cold surfaces or volatile liquids.[9,47,48] Liquid propane boils at −47.2F (−44°C) and is stored in pressurized tanks that can leak or spray. The propane rapidly vaporizes on warm skin producing a severe evaporative freeze injury. This injury has an appearance similar to a deep scald,[46,48] but will not cause the protein denaturation seen with burns. The subcutaneous and muscular edema that develops can be severe, and case reports describe compartment syndrome and severe myonecrosis.[46–49]

Tissue Thawing

The second opportunity for cellular death is during the thawing stage,[30] although the mechanism that

potentiates tissue damage with slow rewarming is unclear.[50] The existing data, derived from different animal models with variable warming protocols, are difficult to interpret. Injury models include air cooling,[51] more typical of frostbite, and immersion in −4°F (−20°C) liquid,[52] akin to a flash freeze. These methods create significant differences in the cold injury pathophysiology, making conclusions less meaningful.

Gradual warming has been studied in animal models. As vasospasm relents, vascular flow returns and the tissue thaws from the central blood vessels outward, gradually progressing from proximal to distal.[53,54] Almost immediately, intravascular platelet aggregation occurs in the arterioles, although few neutrophils are seen. Within 60 minutes, the entire microvasculature shows endothelial damage, and leukocyte aggregation is progressive for up to 6 hours post-thaw.[42] If similar studies use rapid rewarming, there is an initial return of blood flow to pre-freeze rates, without vasospasm or clot formation, and capillary flow is maintained (**Fig. 2**). Within 20 minutes, the blood flow becomes sluggish starting in the venules and proceeding retrograde through the capillary bed to the arterioles.[55] With arteriole inflow unchanged, progressive edema appears.[55]

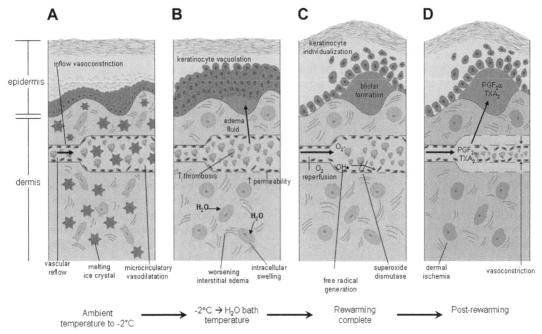

Fig. 2. Tissue thawing. (*A*) Tissue rewarming begins. (*B*) Extracellular ice crystals melt. Freeze-induced endothelial cell disruption promotes development of edema. (*C*) Continued endothelial cell injury occurs from free radicals, whose toxic effect is blocked by SOD. Epidermal blisters may develop. (*D*) PGF$_{2\alpha}$ and TXA$_2$-induced microcirculatory vasoconstriction and platelet aggregation result in worsening dermal ischemia. (*Adapted from* Britt LD, Dascombe WH, Rodriguez A. New horizons in management of hypothermia and frostbite injury. Surg Clin North Am 1991;71(2):361; with permission.)

Once vascular flow returns, the peripheral pulses are bounding and there is increased perfusion, color and capillary refill.[56] Animal studies demonstrate palpable pulses and minimal changes in angiographic flow before 60 minutes post-frostbite.[57] With rapid rewarming techniques, the vascular permeability and edema still result but there is less irreversible damage to the limb.[58,59]

Tissue Reperfusion

Polymorphonuclear leukocytes and mast cells gradually infiltrate the perfused frostbitten skin. These cells and the damaged vascular endothelium release of inflammatory mediators such as prostaglandins, thromboxanes, bradykinin, and histamine.[20,60] Endothelial cells damaged by the freezing process now swell, releasing products from the arachidonic acid cascade[39] and oxygen free radicals.[4,30] An efflux of transcapillary fluid is augmented by endothelial gaps created by the edema.[4] In severe injuries, erythrocyte extravasation and perivascular hemorrhage produce hemorrhagic blisters.[42,44,53,55]

Monoclonal antibodies that prevent leukocyte adherence and aggregation demonstrated beneficial effects in a slow freeze animal model.[61] The administration of a superoxide free radical

scavenger, superoxide dismutase (SOD), reduced the tissue loss in a similar model.[62] SOD did not alter the morphologic changes induced by freezing when tissues were warmed by slow thawing.[42]

The progressive edema causes capillary compression and vascular stasis.[63] The cold-injured endothelial cells can detach from the basement membrane of small and large vessels and occlude the distal capillary beds, completing the "double vascular lesion."[31,62] The denuded basement membrane is thrombogenic and thrombosis can occur in the stagnant column of blood. In a rabbit model designed to produce a fourth-degree injury, the spasm was progressive and peaked at approximately 48 hours after injury.[57] These occlusions of the arteries and arterioles result in the characteristic "glovelike" distribution of necrosis seen late in severe frostbite.[64] This progressive ischemic injury may be aggravated by a lack of nitric oxide production from the damaged endothelium.[65]

The hallmark of significant frostbite is blister formation. Vesicles form 6 to 24 hours after rewarming as blood flows into the area and extravasated fluid accumulates beneath the detached epidermal sheet. Little or no blister fluid accumulation in the severely injured distal tissue implies no blood flow and a poor prognosis. Hemorrhagic blisters indicate disruption of the dermal plexus, which also portends to a less favorable outcome than areas with clear bullae.

Bullae from patients with frostbite of the hands contain high levels of prostaglandin $F_{2\alpha}$ ($PGF_{2\alpha}$) and thromboxane B_2 (metabolite of thromboxane A_2, TXA_2), although having reduced levels of prostaglandin E_2 (PGE_2).[60] $PGF_{2\alpha}$ and TXA_2 produce vasoconstriction, leukocyte adherence, and platelet aggregation. These have been shown to mediate dermal ischemia in burns[66] and pedicle flaps,[60] suggesting a similar process of progressive dermal ischemia. $PGF_{2\alpha}$ is in equilibrium with PGE_2 by the enzyme PGE_2 9-keto-reductase, so as the vasoconstricting prostanoid increases, the vasodilator levels decline.[67]

Immunomodulation

Several agents effective against the arachidonic acid cascade have been tested in frostbite injuries. Aspirin and steroids had some positive effects.[39,68] However, these agents block all arachidonic acid metabolites including prostaglandins beneficial to healing,[60] limiting their attractiveness.[44] Ibuprofen, a specific TXA_2 inhibitor, has been associated with the best tissue salvage, and is currently the standard pharmacologic treatment.[44] Concentrated topical aloe vera gel and oral pentoxifylline were found to improve tissue survival alone or in combination.[40]

CLINICAL MANIFESTATIONS

Frostbite symptoms are predictable and can indicate the severity of the injury. Initially, the patient may describe a feeling of numbness in the affected hands, often accompanied by clumsiness and a lack of fine control. This numbness is replaced by a throbbing sensation on rewarming that may last for days or even weeks. Residual tingling sensations may develop, with occasional electric shock-type sensations, as nerve function returns.[20]

The extent of the frostbite injury is determined by clinical examination and the healing outcome of the injured sites. Frozen skin is cold, white, and firm to the touch.[29] No descriptive or prognostic assessment can be made until the tissues have thawed.[10,69] The older classification defines injury grades first- to fourth-degree (much like thermal burns),[69] but currently most clinicians categorize injuries as either superficial or deep, as advocated by Mills.[70] However attempts at early clinical assessment for tissue viability have poor accuracy,[6,71] and progressive changes in the clinical appearance are expected.[50] Definitive classification may not be possible for 10 days or more.[72]

First-degree frostbite is a superficial injury indicated by the presence of intact sensation, normal-to-hyperemic skin color, and no blister formation on rewarming.[29] The patient may exhibit a mild burning, stinging, or throbbing which is transient. Hyperhidrosis may result, and the involved skin will undergo a more rapid turnover exemplified by desquamation.[31] There is no tissue loss.

Second-degree frostbite is the other superficial injury, and is characterized by clear or milky vesicle formation which will slough and leave viable but painful dermis. Edema formation is common and may be substantial.[31] If the dermis is protected from desiccation or infection, healing is common. The late symptoms are similar to first-degree frostbite.

Third-degree frostbite is a deep injury that results in hemorrhagic blisters indicating subdermal plexus destruction.[44] These blisters are typically smaller but located deeper in the dermis, and are located more proximal on the extremity.[69] The skin is violaceous, soft, or boggy, and does not blanch to palpation.[29] Initially there is no sensation but later progresses to shooting, throbbing, and burning pain sensations.[31] Paresthesia and causalgia are common.

Fourth-degree frostbite results in a mottled, cyanotic skin appearance.[31] The depth of necrosis involves deeper structures such as muscle and bone.[29,30] Edema forms proximal to the involved areas, but not distal. This edema will become the line of demarcation between viable tissue and full-thickness infarction. The distal parts will undergo mummification over a period of weeks (**Fig. 3**).[31,44] The symptoms of third-degree frostbite affect the proximal limb, while numbness persists in the infarcted areas. Neuropathic pain is common after amputation of the mummified digits.

Superficial frostbite includes first- and second-degree injuries, which have an excellent prognosis for recovery. Good prognostic indicators include clear blisters located distally on warm hyperemic limbs with intact sensation. Deep frostbite includes third- and fourth-degree injuries, which are associated with tissue loss and chronic disability. Signs indicating a poor prognosis are hemorrhagic blebs proximally located on the limb, with distal tissue that remains cold, ischemic, and insensate.

TREATMENT
Historical

Larrey recommended friction massage of the frostbitten part with snow, and noted the

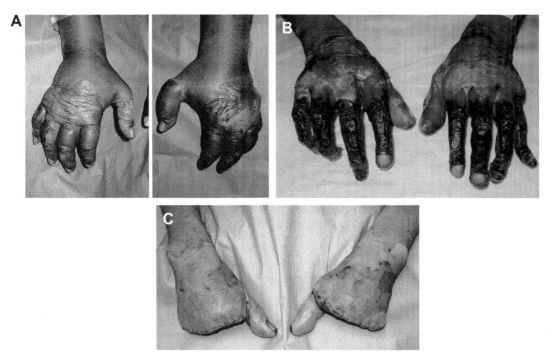

Fig. 3. (*A*) Appearance of a patient with severe frostbite to the hands who presented more than 24 hours after injury with prolonged warm ischemia; not qualifying for thrombolytic therapy. Note the hemorrhagic blebs on both hands. (*B*) Appearance of the eventual mummification of this patient's second through fifth fingers on both hands. (*C*) This patient was able to retain his thumbs.

similarities between the appearance of reperfused frostbite and burns. He recognized that warming the affected area next to a campfire initially improved the color of the frozen limb, but realized the edema (and sometimes a superimposed burn) that resulted was detrimental, and that the cycle of freeze-thaw-freeze was devastating.[20] Although rubbing snow on a frostbitten part would eventually be discredited, the dictum to avoid thawing until definitive rewarming can be accomplished persists today.[4,9,10,29]

The treatment of frostbite remained essentially unchanged for more than 140 years.[20] In the 1930s, research at the Kirov Institute in Leningrad disputed the belief that rapid warming of frostbite was harmful. Using a rabbit ear model, better tissue viability was achieved with active warming techniques (warm water) than by slow warming (rubbing with snow).[73] The publication was in Russian and went undiscovered by Western scientists for another decade.

Scientists at Stanford University were invited by the US government to devise a model and treatment plan for trench foot. They developed a model that was more appropriate for studying frostbite. Their subsequent experiments elucidated much of what we understand today about local cold injuries.[7] Hamill is credited with the first rapid rewarming of a patient with frostbite and hypothermia.[70] This landmark work has become the foundation of frostbite treatment today.[20]

Hypothermia

Severe frostbite may jeopardize one or more limbs, but it is rarely life threatening, with mortality rates less than 3%.[74] Hypothermia can be lethal and must be treated as the top priority.[75] Continuous core temperature monitoring is imperative; a Foley catheter with a built-in thermostat probe is optimal and readily available. Truncal immersion in water at 104°F (40°C) will rapidly correct mild to moderate hypothermia. When core temperature reaches 95°F (35°C), immersion of a single extremity at a time is performed.[29] If the extremities are submerged before core rewarming, the patient may experience "afterdrop," as the cold peripheral blood returns to the core and causes the central temperature to plummet. If the returning blood is acidic and high in potassium, cardiac dysrhythmia and vascular collapse may result, known as "rewarming shock."[50,75] Other methods to achieve rapid rewarming of hypothermic patients exist but are beyond the scope of this article.

Pre-hospital Care

Frostbite victims are encouraged to never thaw affected tissue in the field.[9] Once thawing has occurred, blisters will form and ambulation will become impossible due to incapacitating pain.[29] Warming affected areas next to a campfire can also induce a thermal burn.[9,28] Wrapping the affected part in a blanket for mechanical protection will minimize further cooling and is the best preparation for transporting a patient with frostbite of the extremities.[4] Transport to emergency services should not be delayed.[10]

There are anecdotal reports of frostbite victims using their frostbitten hands and feet to seek safety, but this may cause additional damage to the frozen tissue.[4,73] For someone stranded alone, the risk may be appropriate if the alternative is becoming 1 of the 650 deaths per year caused by hypothermia.[50]

Hospital Care

The direct injuries caused by tissue crystallization are not correctable. The treatment protocol should be directed at melting the ice crystals, re-establishing blood flow to the affected areas, modulation of the inflammatory cascade that creates reperfusion injury, and correction of the secondary thrombotic processes described above.

The standard initial treatment is rapid rewarming in a 104 to 108°F (40–42°C) water bath for 15 to 30 minutes.[4,39,58] This narrow temperature range is most beneficial[59] and causes the least damage to frozen tissue.[39,44,59] Successful rewarming is often demonstrated by pronounced hyperemia of the affected part.[10,29,31] This coincides with extreme pain in three-quarters of the patients,[44] and requires parenteral narcotic administration.[29,44]

Tertiary Care

The goals of post-thaw treatment are to preserve viable tissue and prevent infection.[31] The classic treatment protocol was published by Robson and Heggers at the University of Chicago in 1983.[39] Most of the components have remained unchanged, and are presented in **Box 2**.[4,29,31,39,44]

After thawing, patients with significant frostbite are admitted to the hospital for pain management, protection, and elevation of the affected areas, and to ensure the proper dressing cares. Physical and occupational therapy are started as the edema resolves. Tetanus prophylaxis is updated according to the ACS guideline for a tetanus-prone wound (repeat if more than 5 years since the last booster). McCauley recounts that tetanus killed thousands of Napoleon's troops who invaded Russia, and as recently as 1985 a frostbite patient developed clinical tetanus.[44]

Any tobacco use can further compromise distal perfusion. A single study found that short-term use

---

Box 2
Standard treatment protocol for frostbite

Admit to the hospital

Rapid rewarming with water at 104 to 108 °F (40–42 °C)

Tetanus prophylaxis (ACS tetanus-prone wound class)

Narcotic analgesics

Ibuprofen (400 mg every 12 hours vs 12 mg/kg/d)

Antibiotics (routine penicillin vs as indicated)

Topical aloe vera every 6 hours (optional)

Limb elevation with splinting as needed

No ambulation until edema has resolved (and only in protective footwear)

No smoking

Daily hydrotherapy

ACS, American College of Surgeons.

---

of a nicotine patch enhances the acute endogenous fibrinolytic capacity in healthy volunteers without changes in vasodilation.[76] Use of transdermal nicotine may be less deleterious than smoking, and has the benefit of keeping patients inside the hospital and warm.

The usefulness of prophylactic antibiotics and the optimal treatment of blisters are debated. Scheduled antibiotics have been advocated to combat the perceived high risk of infection after a local cold injury. Penicillin has been recommended because the edema inactivates the normal bacteriocidal properties of the skin.[44] This is given for 24 to 72 hours after thawing, or until the edema resolves.[31,44,67] Others have argued that the incidence of infection is low (13%), and half of all infected patients present greater than 24 hours post injury with active cellulitis.[13] The authors, and many other clinicians, reserve antibiotics to treat clinical infections.[8,29]

The rationale to debride frostbite blisters is based on findings of high levels of $PGF_{2\alpha}$ and TXA_2 in blister fluid.[60] These arachidonate metabolites were previously shown to be the primary mediators of progressive dermal ischemia in thermal injuries.[77] The belief that these modulators would continue to stimulate the inflammatory process is the basis for aspirating[29] or debriding[31,44,67] these blisters. Although some clinicians debride all blisters,[4] others argue that hemorrhagic blisters result from dermal plexus destruction and debridement risks further damage the tenuous microvascular network.[27] Experimental and clinical data demonstrate better tissue healing when using protocols that include ibuprofen and topical aloe vera, but no studies have been done to determine if blister aspiration is beneficial in patients receiving systemic antiprostanoids and topical antithromboxane preparations. The authors find removal of blister fluid scientifically sound, and the deflated blisters temporarily prevent desiccation of the damaged dermal bed.

ADJUNCTIVE THERAPIES
Thrombolytics

The standard treatment of severe frostbite is directed at melting the extracellular ice crystals without causing thermal injury, returning blood flow to the affected area, and modifying the inflammatory response. The authors believe a major determinant of outcome is the microvascular thrombosis that occurs after rewarming.[20,29,30,44,50] The combination of rapid rewarming, oral ibuprofen, and topical aloe vera treatment attempt to decrease this process,[27,44] but have only been modestly successful. Thrombolytics are conceptually attractive because they potentially correct the pathology leading to delayed tissue necrosis.

An animal study showed that intra-arterial (IA) urokinase resulted in less tissue loss compared with slow rewarming but was not better than rapid rewarming.[78] Sirr described the first use of IA tissue plasminogen activator (tPA) in four patients in 1992.[79] The investigators subsequently published their 14-year series using tPA on 19 patients (6 IA and 13 intravenous). They had restrictive inclusion criteria and used technetium (Tc)-99m 3-phase bone scan on admission to predict tissue viability. Of the 174 digits determined on bone scan to be at risk, only 33 digits ultimately required amputation. Using a modified version of our treatment protocol, Bruen and colleagues from Salt Lake City evaluated 32 frostbite patients, and six received IA tPA for angiographically documented arterial occlusions. The rate of digit salvage was 90% compared with 59% without this intervention.[22]

At Regions Burn Center, the authors have selectively used angiography and IA thrombolytics since 1994 (**Fig. 4**). The lytic agents have included urokinase, tPA, reteplase, and tenecteplase at different times, depending on their commercial availability. Our inclusion criteria are more inclusive than the two cited reports, and the authors have attempted lytic therapy for persons up to 24 hours post-rewarming (warm

ischemic time). The authors obtained complete vascular reperfusion after thrombolytics (demonstrated by angiography) in approximately two-thirds of patients, which was associated with a 98% digit salvage rate. Overall, 83% had at least partial response, as indicated by vascular flow beyond the next joint level. For patients with frostbite of the hands, this partial response resulted in the salvage of 86 joints in nine patients.[26] Our combined experience with thrombolytic therapy shows approximately 75% digit salvage rate for severe frostbite with perfusion deficits (**Table 2**).

Sympathectomy

Acute surgical sympathectomy has been undertaken for frostbite, but was found to increase edema when performed immediately, whereas some edema resolution is noted when performed 24 to 48 hours after thawing.[80] A clinical trial used chemical sympathectomy with reserpine starting within 3 hours of rewarming, and early surgical sympathectomy an average of 3 days later. There was no pain reduction, resolution of edema, or improved tissue preservation. Protection from recurrent cold injury was the only benefit noted.[81] A distal sympathectomy, performed at the level of the individual digital vessels, can alleviate chronic vasospasm following frostbite. In a series of 3 patients, the pain improved, the skin temperature rose by 1.5 to 2.5°C, and their chronic ulcers healed.[82] The increase in temperature is similar to results using biofeedback.[83] These treatments can be beneficial for well selected patients.

Hyperbaric Oxygen

The first use of hyperbaric oxygen (HBO) for frostbite was documented by Ledingham in 1963.[84] Purported benefits include bacteriostasis, decreased edema in post-ischemic tissues, and increased erythrocyte flexibility.[44] A study in healthy volunteers demonstrated vasoconstriction and decreased blood flow with HBO treatment.[20] Anecdotal case reports describe improvement with HBO starting 5 to 10 days post injury,[85,86] a long time frame to begin treatment of impaired microvascular perfusion. In the absence of controlled clinical trials, it is hard to recommend transfer to a facility for an unproven modality.

Other Treatment Modalities

Clinical protocols to maintain blood flow with heparin, warfarin, or dextran have not proved reliable and have largely been abandoned.[10,20]

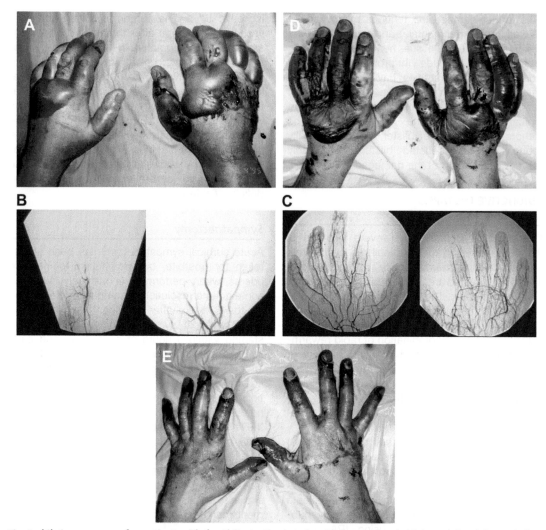

Fig. 4. (*A*) Appearance of a patient with frostbite to the hands with hemorrhagic blebs on the right and clear blebs on the left. (*B*) The patient's angiogram on hospital day number 1 (HD #1) shows no flow to the palmar arch on the right and no flow past the wrist on the left. (*C*) On HD #4, after lytic therapy was complete, the final angiogram shows distal blush on thumb and the third through fifth fingers on both hands, and flow to the distal interphalangeal joint on both indices. (*D*) Appearance of the hands after completion of thrombolytic therapy. (*E*) Weeks later, the patient's hands show good healing. This patient did not require any amputations.

DIAGNOSIS
Bone Scan

[99m]Tc pertechnetate scintigraphy can be used to evaluate perfusion of bone and soft tissues. These studies reveal flow in three phases: early blood, early bone, and late bone. The lack of flow in the late (bone) phase is a poor prognostic sign of tissue healing with extremity frostbite. The predictive accuracy of the scans varies with time post injury.[87–90] Several reports have found good correlation with final surgical outcomes,[89,90] similar to early animal models.[91] The diagnostic accuracy 48 hours post injury is only 84%, but repeat scans at 7 to 10 days are more accurate.[90] Cauchy and

colleagues recommend scanning at 48 hours and again at 8 days post-rewarming.[92] Bhatnagar and colleagues have found that absence of uptake for even the first 10 days does not always lead to tissue infarction.[72] The authors do not obtain bone scans in frostbite patients because the results are erratic. Allowing 2 to 3 weeks for the vascular instability to resolve before recommending amputation seems prudent, especially for the upper extremities.[44]

Nuclear Medicine Studies

There is a single report of two frostbite patients in whom MRI and magnetic resonance angiography

Table 2
Thrombolytic outcomes across three burn centers

Burn Center	Number of Patients	Digits at Risk (Hands & Feet)	Number of Amputations	Percent Requiring Amputations
Salt Lake City[a]	6	59	6	10
Minneapolis[b]	19	174	33	19
St. Paul[c]	66	482	148	31
Overall	91	715	187	26

[a] *Data from* Bruen KJ, Ballard JR, Morris SE, et al. Reduction of the incidence of amputation in frostbite injury with thrombolytic therapy. Arch Surg 2007;142:546–53.
[b] *Data from* Twomey JA, Peltier GL, Zera RT. An open-label study to evaluate the safety and efficacy of tissue plasminogen activator in treatment of severe frostbite. J Trauma 2005;59:1350–5.
[c] *Data from* Jenabzadeh K, Mohr WJ, Ahernholz DH. Frostbite: a single institution's twenty year experience with intra-arterial thrombolytic therapy. J Burn Care Res 2009;30(2):S103.

(MRA) were compared with ^{99m}Tc bone scans. Both patients had proximal vascular occlusions at the ankle and mid-hand. MRI/MRA allowed better visualization of the occluded vessels, but both studies indicated the same anatomic site for amputation. Digits have limited soft tissue, which may impair the quality of MRI/MRA imaging of frostbitten hands.[20]

DEFINITIVE SURGICAL MANAGEMENT

Urgent surgical intervention for local cold injuries is unusual, but necessary on occasion for soft tissue infections not controlled by antibiotics.[50] The authors use a guillotine amputation as the primary procedure, followed by secondary closure when the infection is controlled. Despite the potential for significant edema formation following rewarming, compartment syndrome is rare, occurring in less than 1% of our patients.[26]

The traditional surgical adage for frostbite, "frostbite in January, amputation in July," is no longer valid. The risk of infection, loss of functional hand use, and psychological hardship associated with many months of watching the mummification process is no longer necessary.[30] Fourth-degree frostbite forms hard, black eschar starting 2 weeks post injury,[30] and clinical demarcation with mummified digits usually occurs by 3 to 4 weeks post injury.[44] Surgical interventions can then be performed in most patients.

Early Surgical Management

Advocates of early surgery state that the results of the bone scans are descriptive enough to guide early surgical interventions. The most aggressive attempt at tissue salvage has been undertaken at the University of Chicago. They used a standardized protocol of rapid rewarming and local cares as discussed earlier. At 48 hours, they obtained an initial bone scan to assess tissue perfusion to the affected areas. If there were abnormalities in the perfusion, they repeated the study 72 hours later. For persistent deficits in the delayed bone phase, they performed surgical excision of nonperfused soft tissues by post injury day 10 and covered the remaining tendons, nerves, and bone with a myocutaneous flap. They reported that follow-up bone scans showed normal resumption of bone and soft tissue perfusion.[30,93] This treatment algorithm limited the extent of amputations in selected patients, the long-term functional results have not been published.

SURGICAL CAVEATS

As with most debilitating conditions, frostbite of the hands should be treated by a multidisciplinary team, including a burn surgeon, a hand surgeon, a physical medicine and rehabilitation specialist, and an occupational-hand therapist. The functional rehabilitation of the frostbitten hands can be optimized using this team approach. If amputations are required, discussions regarding the level of amputation among the team are appropriate to provide the patient with the best outcome. The following reflects an approach recommended by our rehabilitation physiatrist and our plastic-hand surgeon. (S.V. Fisher and L.K. Kalliainen, personal communication, February 2009.)

Rehabilitation Specialist's Perspective

From a rehabilitative and functional standpoint, 80% to 85% of the activities of daily living (ADL) using the hands rely on proprioception, not the length or strength of the remaining digits. The "eyes of the hand" are the thumb, index, and middle finger, and they require sensation to have peak functionality. Our goal in rehabilitating patients with frostbite injuries to the hands is for them to be independent in their usual ADL, such as dressing, grooming, eating, and writing.

Frostbite patients can be disabled because of the loss of proprioception. Saving digit length (ie, middle and distal phalanges) in the frostbitten hand is a mistake. The decision at which level an amputation is to be performed should based on the ultimate functionality of the digit, not its length. Although it is ideal to salvage length without compromising soft tissue coverage, in most cases it is preferable to perform amputations in the hand more proximally. This procedure will allow more soft tissue coverage,[94] avoid tension, and will have the surgical scar situated dorsally. These considerations will help diminish the pain factor post-amputation and maximize proprioception. Maintaining sensation to the distal soft tissue is paramount to the functionality of the hand.

If transmetacarpal amputation is required, enough bone should be resected to allow for adequate soft tissue coverage without tension. If a hand prosthesis is anticipated, the patient would benefit most by having a thicker soft tissue flap to cover a more proximal transmetacarpal amputation. This procedure will facilitate a more comfortable fitting of the hand prosthesis.

Surgeon's Perspective

Avoid skin grafts if possible, as it increases cold intolerance and results in decreased sensibility. Retain length without stretching the soft tissue envelope tightly over the end of the bone. Preserving length is plausible if the skin has sloughed but the underlying tissues are viable. A negative pressure wound dressing can be used in those circumstances to avoid desiccation and prepare for a local or free tissue transfer.[93,95,96] For patients with a shortened thumb and index finger due to frostbite, a thumb and index finger web space deepening procedure has been used at our center. This procedure maintains some of the opposability, pinch, and grip capability of the thumb.[97–99]

For the second through fourth fingers, complete amputation of the proximal phalanx should be avoided if possible.[4] Maintaining as much length as possible on the index finger, without violating the above tenets, allows the patient to maintain some grip and pinch function. Conversely, leaving only a small piece of the proximal phalanx on the fifth finger should be avoided, as it frequently is hooked on pockets, causes discomfort when trying to write, and is cosmetically unappealing.

PROGNOSIS AND SEQUELAE

Frostbitten tissues seldom recover completely.[50] Long-term symptoms include cold sensitivity (75%), sensory loss (68%), hyperhidrosis (75%), and chronic pain (67%).[100] Patients with tissue loss almost uniformly report an electric shock-type of pain.[44] Osteoarthritis develops in approximately half of the hands with frostbite involvement,[21,31] 38% report joint problems, and heterotopic calcification can occur.[20] Benign skin color changes are common (56%).[100] There is a single report of a Marjolin ulcer developing 60 years after frostbite of the foot.[101]

Children have an increased potential for bony abnormalities following frostbite, even without initial soft tissue loss.[30] Freezing damages the

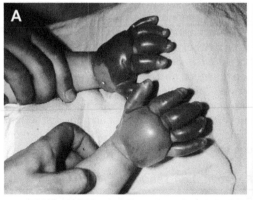
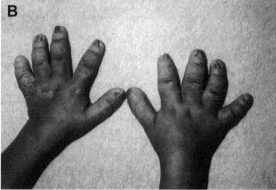

Fig. 5. (*A*) Appearance 6 hours after a frostbite injury in a 3-year-old child. (*B*) Appearance 3 years after injury. Note impaired bone growth in the digits. (*From* Ahrenholz DH. Frostbite. Problems Gen Surg 2003;20(1): 135; with permission.)

articular cartilage,[73] although the radiographic changes appear 6 to 12 months later.[4] The articular surface may be completely replaced by scar tissue.[53] The visible deformities (**Fig. 5**) include dwarfing of the middle and distal phalanges, degenerative arthritis, and malalignment of the proximal and distal interphalangeal joints. These joints are more lax and the skin is loose,[4] although the more proximal joints, including the metacarpal phalangeal joints and wrist, are spared.[102] Bony growth arrest with shortening has been reported if the epiphyseal plates are damaged.[103]

SUMMARY

The cold has been a lethal adversary throughout history. Our ability to live beyond our tropical thermal comfort zone is due to planning and protection against the elements. Any impairment in our mental capacity, judgment, or risk taking behavior can put us at odds with our environment. The most frequent factors related to frostbite injury are alcohol and drugs, mental illness, and lack of available shelter.

Frostbite results in direct and indirect mechanisms of tissue injury. The direct process occurs when ice crystals form in the tissues at temperatures below 28.4°F ($-2°C$). Although this results in little permanent damage, it creates a larger obstacle during tissue rewarming. It is universally recognized that rapid warming in water at 104 to 108°F (40 to 42°C) is the most effective initial treatment of frostbite, but as many as half of all frostbite patients have thawed to room temperatures before receiving any medical care. Rapid rewarming restores blood flow to the distal extremities, ischemic from the persistent vasoconstriction caused during the freezing process. The damaged tissue releases inflammatory mediators in the form of $PGF_{2\alpha}$ and TXA_2, which induces permeability of the capillary membranes; significant edema results further jeopardizing the tissues. Agents to block components of the arachidonic acid cascade have been used in combination with rapid rewarming. Despite these therapies, severe frostbite still causes tissue necrosis and amputations.

The injured endothelium separates and embolizes, leaving a raw vessel surface for platelets aggregation and progressive vascular obstruction. If this thrombosis is limited to some areas of the microcirculation, soft tissue may be lost when the digits survive. If the larger arterioles and arteries are affected, the entire limb is at risk for necrosis. The major determinant of tissue necrosis is the progressive microvascular thrombosis. Thrombolytics have been used at several northern burn centers with documented return of blood flow in previously thrombosed vessels. The combined digit salvage rate has been 75%.

Frostbite therapies have the laudable goal of avoiding amputation. Our patients appreciate these efforts, but must deal with the common problems of pain, sensory loss, hyperhidrosis, and degenerative arthritis. Better methods to prevent these debilitating long-term sequelae are required. Salvaging a digit or hand, only to have life-long chronic pain, may be a hollow victory for the patient.

ACKNOWLEDGMENTS

Stephen V. Fisher, MD (Physical Medicine and Rehabilitation Specialist), Loree K. Kalliainen, MD (Plastic and Hand Surgeon), Frederick W. Endorf, MD (Burn, Trauma and Critical Care), and the Department of Plastic and Hand Surgery at Regions Hospital (St. Paul, MN, USA).

REFERENCES

1. Bangs CC. Hypothermia and frostbite. Emerg Med Clin North Am 1984;2:475–87.
2. Post PW, Donner DD. Frostbite in a pre-Columbian mummy. Am J Phys Anthropol 1972;37:187–91.
3. Chadwick J. The medical works of Hippocrates. Oxford: Blackwell Scientific Publications; 1950.
4. Vogel JE, Dellon AL. Frostbite injuries of the hand. Clin Plast Surg 1989;16(3):565–76.
5. Larrey DJ. Memoirs of military surgery and campaigns of the French armies. Baltimore (MD): Cushing; 1814.
6. O'Sullivan ST, O'Shaughnessy M, O'Connor TPF. Baron Larrey and cold injury during the campaigns of Napoleon. Ann Plast Surg 1995;34(4):446–9.
7. Paton BC. A history of frostbite treatment. Int J Circumpolar Health 2000;59(2):99–107.
8. Petrone P, Kuncir E, Asensio JA. Surgical management and strategies in the treatment of hypothermia and cold injury. Emerg Med Clin North Am 2003;21: 1165–78.
9. Purdue GF, Hunt JL. Cold injury: a collective review. J Burn Care Rehabil 1986;7(4):331–42.
10. Reamy BV. Frostbite: review and current concepts. J Am Board Fam Pract 1998;11(1):34–40.
11. Miller BJ, Chasmar LR. Frostbite in Saskatoon: a review of 10 winters. Can J Surg 1980;23(5):423–6.
12. Pinzur MS, Weaver FM. Is urban frostbite a psychiatric disorder? Orthopedics 1997;20(1):43–5.
13. Urschel J. Frostbite: predisposing factors and predictors of poor outcome. J Trauma 1990;30(3): 340–3.
14. Valnicek SM, Chasmar LR, Clapson JB. Frostbite in the prairies: a 12-year review. Plast Reconstr Surg 1993;92(4):633–41.

15. Ervasti O, Hassi J, Rintamaki H, et al. Sequelae of moderate finger frostbite as assessed by subjective sensations, clinical signs, and thermophysiological responses. Int J Circumpolar Health 2000; 59(2):137–45.

16. Pichotka J, Lewis RB. Use of heparin in treatment of experimental frostbite. Proc Soc Exp Biol Med 1949;72(1):130–6.

17. Bracker MD. Environmental and thermal injury. Clin Sports Med 1992;11(2):419–36.

18. Christenson C, Stewart C. Frostbite. Am Fam Physician 1984;30(6):111–22.

19. Dalton J, Robertson M. Cold injury caused by psychiatric illness: six case reports. Br J Psychiatry 1982;140:615–8.

20. Murphy J, Banwell P, Roberts A, et al. Frostbite: pathogenesis and treatment. J Trauma 2000; 48(1):171–89.

21. McKendry RJ. Frostbite arthritis. Can Med Assoc J 1981;125(10):1128–30.

22. Bruen KJ, Ballard JR, Morris SE, et al. Reduction of the incidence of amputation in frostbite injury with thrombolytic therapy. Arch Surg 2007;142: 546–53.

23. Kyosola K. Clinical experiences in the management of cold injuries: a study of 110 cases. J Trauma 1974;14(1):32–6.

24. Antti-Poika I, Pohjolainen T, Alaranta H. Severe frostbite of the upper extremities - a psychosocial problem mostly associated with alcohol abuse. Scand J Soc Med 1990;18(1):59–61.

25. Ozyazgan I, Irfan M, Melli M, et al. Eicosanoids and inflammatory cells in frostbitten tissue: prostacyclin, thromboxane, polymorphonuclear leukocytes, and mast cells. Plast Reconstr Surg 1998;101(7): 1881–6.

26. Jenabzadeh K, Mohr WJ, Ahernholz DH. Frostbite: a single institution's twenty year experience with intra-arterial thrombolytic therapy [abstract]. J Burn Care Res 2009;30(2):S103.

27. McCauley RL, Heggers JP, Robson MC. Frostbite: methods to minimize tissue loss. Postgrad Med 1990;88(8):67–77.

28. Ahrenholz DH, Solem LD. Frostbite. In: Copeland EM, Howard RJ, Warshaw AJ, et al, editors. Current practice of surgery. New York: Churchill Livingstone; 1993. p. 1–11.

29. Ahrenholz DH. Frostbite. Problems in General Surgery 2003;20(1):129–37.

30. Su CW, Lohman R, Gottlieb LJ. Frostbite of the upper extremity. Hand Clin 2000;16(2):235–47.

31. Britt LD, Dascombe WH, Rodriguez A. New horizons in management of hypothermia and frostbite injury. Surg Clin North Am 1991;71(2):345–70.

32. Rustin MH, Newton JA, Smith NP, et al. The treatment of chilblains with nifedipine: the results of a pilot study, a double-blind placebo-controlled randomized study and a long-term open trial. Br J Dermatol 1989;120(2):267–75.

33. Stewart C. Regulation of Heat Gain and Loss: Beyond the Road, Environmental Emergencies for Emergency Service Providers. Charles Stewart and Associates, 1994.

34. Holm PC, Vanggaard L. Frostbite. Plast Reconstr Surg 1974;54(5):544–51.

35. Burton AC. Physiology of cutaneous circulation, thermoregulatory functions. In: Rothman S, editor. The human integument. Washington, DC: American Association for the Advancement of Science; 1959. p. 77–88.

36. Guyton AC. Textbook of medical physiology. 8th edition. Philadelphia: WB Saunders; 1991.

37. Rintamaki H. Human responses to cold. Ala Med 2007;49(2 Suppl):29–31.

38. Dana AS, Rex IH, Samitz MH. The hunting reaction. Arch Dermatol 1969;99:441–50.

39. McCauley RL, Hing DN, Robson MC, et al. Frostbite injuries: a rational approach based on the pathophysiology. J Trauma 1983;23(2):143–7.

40. Miller MB, Koltai PJ. Treatment of experimental frostbite with pentoxifylline and aloe vera cream. Arch Otolaryngol Head Neck Surg 1995;121(6): 678–80.

41. Lang K, Weiner D, Boyd LJ. Frostbite: physiology, pathology and therapy. N Engl J Med 1947;237: 383–9.

42. Marzella LM, Jesudass RR, Manson PN. Morphologic characterization of acute injury to vascular endothelium of skin after frostbite. Plast Reconstr Surg 1989;83:67–75.

43. Wilson O, Goldman RF. Role of air temperature and wind in the time necessary for a finger to freeze. J Appl Phys 1970;29(5):658–64.

44. McCauley RL, Killyon GW, Smith DJ, et al. Frostbite. In: Auerback, editor. Wilderness medicine. 5th edition. Philadelphia: Mosby Elsevier; 2007. p. 195–210.

45. Dinep M. A review of current theories and their application to treatment. Conn Med 1975;39: 8–10.

46. Hicks LM, Hunt JL, Baxter CR. Liquid propane injury: a clinicopathologic and experimental study. J Trauma 1979;19:701–3.

47. Corn CC, Wachtel TL, Malone JM, et al. Liquid-propane freeze injury: a case history. J Burn Care Rehabil 1991;12(2):136–40.

48. Matook GM, Sasken H, Akelman E. Propane thermal injuries: case report and review of the literature. J Trauma 1994;37(2):318–21.

49. Corn CC, Malone JM, Wachtel TL, et al. The protection against and treatment of a liquid propane freeze injury: an experimental model. J Burn Care Rehabil 1991;12(3):516–20.

50. Jurkovich GJ. Environmental cold-induced injury. Surg Clin North Am 2007;87(1):247–67.

51. Schoning P, Hall SM, Hamlet MP. Experimental frostbite: freezing times, rewarming times, and lowest temperatures of pig skin exposed to chilled air. Cryobiology 1990;27(2):189–93.

52. Weatherley-White RC, Knize DM, Geisterfer DJ, et al. Experimental studies in cold injury. V. Circulatory hemodynamics. Surgery 1969;66(1):208–14.

53. Bigelow DR, Ritchie GW. The effects of frostbite in childhood. J Bone Joint Surg Am 1963;45(B):122–31.

54. Fuhrman FA, Crismon JM. Studies on gangrene following cold injury. General course of events in rabbit feet and ears following untreated cold injury. J Clin Invest 1947;26(2):236–44.

55. Bourne MH, Piepkorn MW, Clayton F, et al. Analysis of microvascular changes in frostbite injury. J Surg Res 1986;40(1):26–35.

56. Pirozynski WJ, Webster DR. Redistribution of K and Na in experimental frostbite. Surg Forum 1953;3:665–70.

57. Lazarus HM, Hutto W. Electric burns and frostbite: patterns of vascular injury. J Trauma 1982;22(7):581–5.

58. Mills WJ. Frostbite: a method of management including rapid thawing. Northwest Med 1966;65(2):119–25.

59. Fuhrman FA, Crismon JM. Studies on gangrene following cold injury. Treatment of cold injury by means of immediate rapid rewarming. J Clin Invest 1947;26(3):476–85.

60. Robson MC, Heggers JP. Evaluation of hand frostbite blister fluid as a clue to pathogenesis. J Hand Surg 1981;6(1):43–7.

61. Mileski WJ, Raymond JF, Winn RK, et al. Inhibition of leukocyte adherence and aggregation for treatment of severe cold injury in rabbits. J Appl Phys 1993;74:1432–6.

62. Manson PN, Jesudass R, Marzella L, et al. Evidence for an early free radical-mediated reperfusion injury in frostbite. Free Radic Biol Med 1991;10(1):7–11.

63. Crismon JM, Fuhrman FA. Studies on gangrene following cold injury. VIII. The use of casts and pressure dressings in the treatment of severe frostbite. J Clin Invest 1947;26(3):486–96.

64. Davis RG. Amputations in frostbite. Can Med Assoc J 1957;77(10):948–52.

65. Tercan M, Bekerecioglu M. Decreased serum nitric oxide level in experimental frostbite injury: a preliminary study. Ann Plast Surg 2002;48(1):107–8.

66. Heggers JP, Robson MC, Zachary LS. Thromboxane inhibitors for the prevention of progressive dermal ischemia due to the thermal injury. J Burn Care Rehabil 1985;6(6):466–8.

67. Heggers JP, Robson MC, Manavalen K, et al. Experimental and clinical observations on frostbite. Ann Emerg Med 1987;16(9):191–7.

68. Vaughn PB. Local cold injury: menace to military operations, a review. Mil Med 1980;145(5):305–11.

69. Edlich RF, Chang DE, Birk KA, et al. Cold injuries. Compr Ther 1989;15(9):13–21.

70. Mills WJ, Whaley R, Fish W. Frostbite: experience with rapid rewarming and ultrasonic therapy: Part III. 1961. Ala Med 1993;35(1):28–35.

71. Orr KD, Fainer DC. Cold injuries in Korea clinic: the winter of 1950–1951. Medicine 1952;31(1):177.

72. Bhatnagar A, Sarker BB, Sawroop K, et al. Diagnosis, characterisation and evaluation of treatment response of frostbite using pertechnetate scintigraphy: a prospective study. Eur J Nucl Med Mol Imaging 2002;29(2):170–5.

73. Ariev TY. Slow vs. rapid warming of frozen extremities. In: Narkomzdrav, editor. Monograph on frostbite. USSR: SHC; 1939. p. 1–169.

74. Boswick JA. Cold injuries. Major Probl Clin Surg 1976;19:96–106.

75. Wittmers LE. Pathophysiology of cold exposure. Minn Med 2001;84(11):30–6.

76. Pellegrini MP, Newby DE, Maxwell S, et al. Short-term effects of transdermal nicotine on acute tissue plasminogen activator release in vivo in man. Cardiovasc Res 2001;52:321–7.

77. Cera LM, Heggers JP, Robson MC, et al. The therapeutic efficacy of Aloe vera cream (Dermaide aloe) in thermal injuries: two case reports. J Am Anim Hosp Assoc 1980;16(5):768–72.

78. Zdeblick TA, Field GA, Shaffer JW. Treatment of experimental frostbite with urokinase. J Hand Surg 1988;13(6):948–53.

79. Skolnick AA. Early data suggest clot-dissolving drug may help save frostbitten limbs from amputation. J Am Med Assoc 1992;267(15):2008–9.

80. Golding MR. Protection from the early and late sequelae of frostbite by regional sympathectomy: mechanisms of "cold sensitivity" following frostbite. Surgery 1963;53:303–8.

81. Bouwman DL, Morrison S, Lucas CE, et al. Early sympathetic blockade for frostbite – is it of value? J Trauma 1980;20(9):744–9.

82. Flatt AE. Digital artery sympathectomy. J Hand Surg 1980;5(6):550–6.

83. Brown FE, Jobe JB, Hamlet MP, et al. Induced vasodilation in the treatment of posttraumatic digital cold intolerance. J Hand Surg 1985;11A(3):382–7.

84. Ledingham JGG. Some clinical and experimental applications of high pressure oxygen. Proc R Soc Med 1963;56:999–1002.

85. von Heimburg D, Noah EM, Sieckmann UP, et al. Hyperbaric oxygen treatment in deep frostbite of both hands in a boy. Burns 2001;27(4):404–8.

86. Ward MP, Garnham JR, Simpson BRJ, et al. Frostbite: general observations and report of cases treated by hyperbaric oxygen. Proc R Soc Med 1968;61:33–5.

87. Mehta RC, Wilson MA. Frostbite injury: prediction of tissue viability with triple-phase bone scanning. Radiology 1989;170(2):511–4.

88. Ristkari SK, Vorne M, Mokka RE. Early assessment of amputation level in frostbite by ^{99m}Tc-pertechnetate scan. Case report. Acta Chir Scand 1988; 154(5–6):403–5.

89. Salimi Z, Vas W, Tang-Barton P, et al. Assessment of tissue viability in frostbite by ^{99m}Tc pertechnetate scintigraphy. Am J Roentgenol 1984;142(2):415–9.

90. Cauchy E, Marsigny B, Allamel G, et al. The value of technetium 99 scintigraphy in the prognosis of amputation in severe frostbite injuries of the extremities: a retrospective study of 92 severe frostbite injuries. J Hand Surg 2000;25(5):969–78.

91. Salimi Z, Wolverson MK, Herbold DR, et al. Frostbite: experimental assessment of tissue damage using Tc-99m pyrophosphate. Work in progress. Radiology 1986;161(1):227–31.

92. Cauchy E, Chetaille E, Lefevre M, et al. The role of bone scanning in severe frostbite of the extremities: a retrospective study of 88 cases. Eur J Nucl Med 2000;27(5):497–502.

93. Greenwald D, Cooper B, Gottlieb L. An algorithm for early aggressive treatment of frostbite with limb salvage directed by triple-phase scanning. Plast Reconstr Surg 1998;102(4):1069–74.

94. Louis DS, Lebson PJL, Graham TJ. Amputations. In: Green DP, Hotchkiss RN, Pederson WC, editors. Green's operative hand surgery. 4th edition. New York: Churchill Livingstone; 1999. p. 56–73.

95. House JH, Fidler MO. Frostbite of the hand. In: Green DP, Hotchkiss RN, Pederson WC, editors. Green's operative hand surgery. 4th edition. New York: Churchill Livingstone; 1999. p. 2061–7.

96. Leonard LG, Daane SP, Sellers DS, et al. Salvage of avascular bone from frostbite with free tissue transfer. Ann Plast Surg 2001;46(4):431–3.

97. Kalliainen LK, Schubert W. The management of web space contractures. Clin Plast Surg 2005; 32(4):503–14.

98. Jensen CB, Rayan GM, Davidson R. First web space contracture and hand function. J Hand Surg 1993;18(3):516–20.

99. Sandzen SC. Thumb web reconstruction. Clin Orthop Relat Res 1985;195:66–82.

100. Blair JR, Schatzki R, Orr KD. Sequelae to cold injury in one hundred patients. Follow-up study four years after occurrence of cold injury. J Am Med Assoc 1957;163(14):1203–8.

101. Uysal A, Kocer U, Sungur N, et al. Marjolin's ulcer on frostbite. Burns 2005;31(6):792–4.

102. Carrera GF, Kozin F, Flaherty L, et al. Radiographic changes in the hands following childhood frostbite injury. Skeletal Radiol 1981;6(1):33–7.

103. Selke AC. Destruction of phalangeal epiphyses by frostbite. Radiology 1969;93(4):859–60.

The Use of Skin Substitutes in Hand Burns

Richard Benjamin Lou, MD[a], William L. Hickerson, MD[a,b],*

KEYWORDS

- Hand • Burns • Skin substitute • Bioengineered skin

Eighty percent of patients who have thermal injuries have been reported to have associated hand burns.[1] Due to our hands being are so important in our occupations, activities of daily living, recreational pursuits, as a means of communication, and as part of our overall aesthetic presentation, it is common to see numerous articles regarding hand burns. Although most hand burns that heal within 3 weeks do so without problems, Sheridan showed that 3% of affected patients may still have functional abnormalities. At the other end of the spectrum, in the same study, of those with deep dermal and full-thickness burns requiring surgery, only 81% had normal function and, of those with injuries to the extensor mechanism, joint capsule, or bone, only 9% had normal functional outcomes.[2] As can be seen throughout this issue, the debate continues regarding the timing of excision, the type of excision, the types of grafts used, the depth to take split-thickness skin grafts (STSG), and when or if to use splints or pin fixation.

A skin substitute can be defined as a naturally occurring or synthetic bioengineered product that is used to replace the skin in a temporary or permanent fashion. In this regard an STSG, not containing regenerative capability of hair follicles or sweat glands, would be considered a skin substitute. It seems a moot point therefore whether to consider a skin substitute in those cases that require grafting. On the other hand, questions remain as to how best to obtain skin coverage in the deep hand burn. The purpose of this article is to review the different bioengineered skin substitutes that are available to help minimize the physical impairment and maximize the aesthetic outcomes following thermal injuries to the hand.

The skin is a complicated organ, but its function can be simply described as a protective barrier that has an aesthetic component. Its complexity, however, becomes evident during loss of skin integrity in trauma, burns, or various skin diseases. Many attempts have been made to imitate the structure and function of the skin; yet, despite improving engineering technology and continued efforts, the perfect replacement is still evasive. The ultimate goals following these injuries are, as Pereira notes, to provide rapid coverage while obtaining a functional and durable barrier that will eventually undergo scar maturation and become an aesthetically pleasing unit.[3] Temporary epidermal replacements may be beneficial in superficial to mid-dermal burns, whereas dermal replacements are the primary focus of current skin substitutes that are used for both acute and reconstructive procedures. It has been said that as the epidermis is life and the dermis is the quality of life provided by skin replacements; this is a recurring theme that has been attributed to various investigators, and without the knowledge of the initiator of the statement, more and more investigators agree with the thought process.

[a] Firefighters' Regional Burn Center, 890 Madison Avenue, Suite TG 030, Memphis, TN 38117, USA
[b] Department of Plastic Surgery, University of Tennessee Health Science Center, 890 Madison Avenue, Suite TG 030, Memphis, TN 38117, USA
* Corresponding author. Department of Plastic Surgery, University of Tennessee Health Science Center, 890 Madison Avenue, Suite TG 030, Memphis, TN 38117.
E-mail address: whicker1@utmem.edu (W.L. Hickerson).

Hand Clin 25 (2009) 497–509
doi:10.1016/j.hcl.2009.06.002

BIOENGINEERED PRODUCTS FOR SUPERFICIAL BURN INJURIES
Porcine Products

Several bioengineered products are available for the care of superficial thermal injuries. These products are used to help close the wound, decrease pain, and improve the rate of healing. Throughout the world a variety of xenografts are used as temporary skin substitutes, but porcine grafts are the most common in use today; MediSkin and EZ-Derm (Brennen Medical-LLC, Saint Paul, Minnesota) are the most common porcine products used in the United States. Both products are processed pigskin used for temporary coverage of partial-thickness skin loss or to cover widely meshed autografts.[4] MediSkin, a frozen porcine xenograft, has both dermal and epidermal components and is irradiated to provide sterility. MediSkin is stored at 0°C and has a shelf life of 24 months. EZ-Derm, on the other hand, is a processed dermal porcine graft that is stored at room temperature and has a shelf life of 18 months. Still used early excision and porcine xenografting to treat second-degree burns, which resulted in a decreased length of stay in hospital.[5] The pigskin does not become vascularized and dries with exposure; the resulting stiff cover may limit range of motion during the healing process. It does, however, provide pain control while serving as an epidermal barrier to promote reepithelialization. Of particular note is that some individuals may object to products containing porcine components on religious grounds.[6]

Biobrane

Biobrane (UDL Laboratories Inc., Rockford, Illinois) is a bilaminant skin substitute that was the first biologically based wound dressing approved by the US Food and Drug Administration (FDA) in 1979.[7] Biobrane consists of a nylon mesh bound to silicone; type 1 porcine collagen is covalently bound to the nylon to improve the product's adherence. The silicone is a semipermeable barrier that decreases evaporative losses and serves as an epidermal layer. Full-thickness pores are placed in the product to allow for drainage. Biobrane gloves are available to treat partial-thickness hand burns that have been debrided of all nonviable tissue. Biobrane decreases pain due to its semiocclusive nature, provides direct visualization of the wound bed due to its transparency, and allows improved range of motion as it stretches with movement. If any fluid accumulates beneath the membrane it should be drained and any portion of the glove not adherent to the underlying wound bed should be removed. The glove should be applied using a sterile technique to a wound bed that has been debrided of all nonviable tissue and has been prepared with 1% povidone-iodine, or a similar antiseptic. The fabric should be minimally stretched to remove all wrinkles and secured away from the wound edge. An absorptive dressing followed by a compressive wrap should then be used for 24 to 48 hours.[8] It is important to realize that this is a semiocclusive dressing and if fluid or hematomas accumulate beneath the fabric, infections may occur. The authors either admit the patients overnight to ensure adherence or follow them closely as an outpatient; additionally, an oral first-generation cephalosporin is administered until the product is adherent. Although at one time it was thought that Biobrane increased the risk of infection, Lal and colleagues[9] have shown that in burned children it improves wound healing without an increased risk of infection. After the Biobrane adheres to the wound, no further dressings are required. As the Biobrane becomes loose around the edges it should be trimmed. On reepithelialization of the skin, the Biobrane acquires an opaque appearance, indicating the product is ready for removal. According to a recent study, 69% of the burn units in the United Kingdom use the temporary skin substitute.[10] Demling[11] presented a study including scald injuries to the hand. Collected over a 5-year period, the study showed a significant decrease in healing time, pain, and length of stay, as well as an increase in mobility when Biobrane, as opposed to topical agents, was used to treat superficial 15% to 25% total body surface burns. Again, it needs to be stressed that the key to successfully using Biobrane, or any other bioengineered skin substitute, is to apply the structure to a clean wound bed that is free of infection and any avascular debris (**Figs. 1–3**).

AWBAT

AWBAT (Aubrey Inc., Carlsbad, California) is an advanced next-generation Biobrane that was approved by the FDA in February 2008.[12] Although not clinically available at this writing, the concept is appealing. AWBAT (Advanced Wound Bioengineered Alternative Tissue), with a porosity 500% that of Biobrane, provides an intact three-dimensional nylon structure to improve tissue ingrowth and decrease scarring. The increase in porosity should improve adherence to the wound surface and, coupled with the fact that the type I porcine collagen is mobile rather than covalently bound, it should have no steric hindrance and allow for a more rapid interaction with the fibrin in the wound, allowing a more rapid acute adherence. The

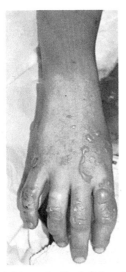

Fig. 1. Superficial burn to the left hand of a 30-year-old woman.

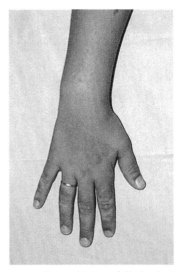

Fig. 3. Four months post injury, fully healed.

increased porosity should also allow for more rapid diffusion of water-soluble antimicrobials. The prototype gloves, available in various sizes for adults and children, should also be easier to apply. They have a 3-year shelf life and do not have any special storage requirements.[13] No clinical data exist at this time comparing Biobrane and AWBAT.

BIOENGINEERED PRODUCTS FOR DEEP HAND BURNS
Allograft

Human cadaver allograft has been the gold standard for temporary skin substitutes. Allograft is preserved in various forms: it comes fresh (refrigerated at 4°C), cryopreserved (frozen at −70°C), lyophilized (freeze-dried), or glycerol preserved. Fresh allograft is often preferred as it is associated with better adherence, rapid revascularization, and better control of microbial growth.[14] May showed that glucose metabolism diminished 10% to 15% a day during refrigeration[15] and, therefore, the allograft is usually cryopreserved within 4 days of harvest unless special techniques are used to maintain viability.[16] Allograft is used to cover extensive partial- and full-thickness wounds, and is a good biologic dressing to cover widely meshed autografts and to cover exfoliative skin disorders. It prevents tissue desiccation, decreases pain, insensible loss of water, electrolytes and protein, suppresses the proliferation of bacteria, and decreases the hypermetabolic component of

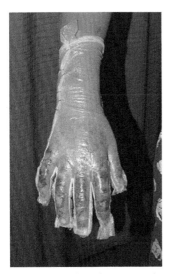

Fig. 2. One week post debridement and application of Biobrane glove.

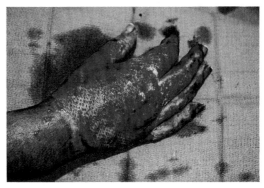

Fig. 4. Right hand of a 16-year-old 2 weeks post burn wound excision and allograft placement. Allograft is well vascularized and ready for tangential excision of the epidermis and placement of sheet graft.

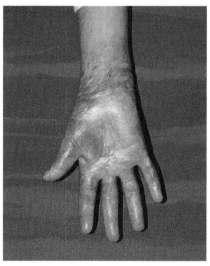

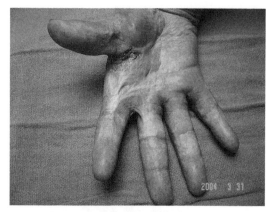

Fig. 7. Long-term follow-up of the same patient grafted with AlloDerm/split-thickness skin grafts. (*Courtesy of* Rajiv Sood, MD, Indianapolis, IN.)

Fig. 5. Right hand of a 42-year-old man with palmar contracture 14 months following burn wound excision and split-thickness skin grafting. (*Courtesy of* Rajiv Sood, MD, Indianapolis, IN.)

thermal injuries.[14] An allograft also serves to prepare the wound bed for future permanent coverage with autografts and can serve as an underlying dermal template on which thin STSG or cultured epidermal autografts may be applied.[17,18] In our experience, the use of allografts in hand burns is most commonly associated with large total body surface burns. Allografts are used as a temporary cover for excised wounds before the application of autografts. If they become engrafted, the epidermis will subsequently be excised and the

allodermis base used as the neodermis for the autograft (**Fig. 4**). This technique has been popularized by Cuono and colleagues[17] for cultured epidermal autografts (CEA) and is based on Medawar's[19] findings that the epidermis and its appendages are the immunogenic elements of skin whereas the dermis, from an immunologic standpoint, is relatively inert. In this case a thinner autograft (0.008–0.010 inches [0.020–0.254 cm]) is appropriate, and this allows more rapid healing and more frequent reharvesting of the donor site. From personal experience, although CEA are rarely used on the hands, the cryopreserved allograft and subsequent thin autograft on the allograft that has had the epidermis excised some 2 to 3 weeks later works exceptionally well (Hickerson, unpublished data, 2008).

AlloDerm

AlloDerm (Life Cell Corporation, Woodlands, Texas) is an acellular dermal matrix engineered from banked, human cadaver skin supplied by

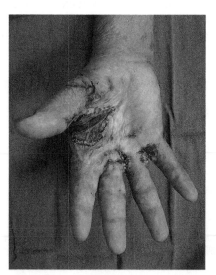

Fig. 6. One week post release of palmar contracture and 1-stage AlloDerm/split-thickness skin graft. (*Courtesy of* Rajiv Sood, MD, Indianapolis, IN.)

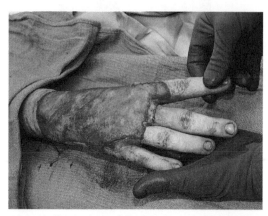

Fig. 8. Well-vascularized Integra at 4 weeks following silicone removal and dermabrasion of the matrix.

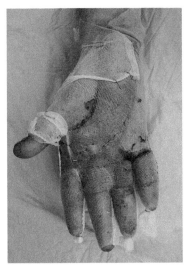

Fig. 9. Biobrane glove used to immobilize the Integra.

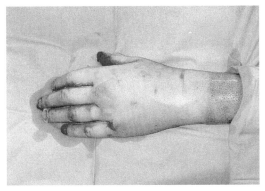

Fig. 11. Deep hand burn in a 63-year-old man. (*Courtesy of* Eric Dantzer, MD, Toulon, France.)

American Association of Tissue Banks (AATB) accredited skin banks. The cadaver skin is chemically treated with an agent to form an inert, deepithelialized acellular dermal matrix, which is then freeze-dried. On rehydration, AlloDerm regenerates into a viable dermis and, when used concurrently with split-thickness skin grafting, can provide a single-stage wound closure. Allo-Derm forms a thick, stable neodermis that aids in decreasing wound contracture rates.[20] A multi-center study in 1996 found that the use of Allo-Derm could greatly reduce donor site morbidity and allow more frequent recropping of donor sites

due to the requirements for a thinner STSG.[21] This is of particular value in large burns when donor site availability is a major issue. In short, AlloDerm potentially would improve functional and cosmetic outcomes in third-degree burns.[22] Bhavsar and Tenenhaus used thin, meshed Allo-Derm to cover exposed joints, tendons, and neurovascular structures in deep hand burns when flaps were not feasible in the acute period. They secured the lateral bands and remnants of the extensor tendons with the acellular dermal matrix and then covered the reconstruction with allografts or Integra, with good soft tissue coverage in 19 of the 26 treated digits.[23] AlloDerm has been in use since 1995. However, its clinical use in burns has been limited at best. Although burn surgeons were initially skeptical of the ability of a dermal substitute to support the vascularization of itself and the overlay autograft, there seems to be an acceptable graft take if the overlying epidermal graft is less than 0.010 (0.0254 cm)

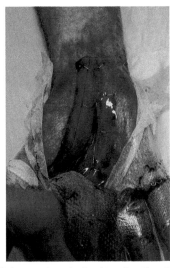

Fig. 10. Biobrane glove incised to visualize the Integra 1 week post application. The Biobrane is then stapled to itself and not totally changed.

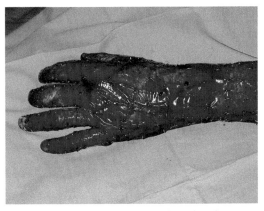

Fig. 12. Acute deep flame burn of the hand in a 63-year-old man. Fascial excision on day four with immediate Integra grafting. (*Courtesy of* Eric Dantzer, MD, Toulon, France.)

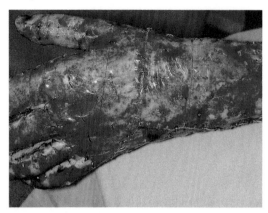

Fig. 13. Integra day 17, same patient. (*Courtesy of* Eric Dantzer, MD, Toulon, France.)

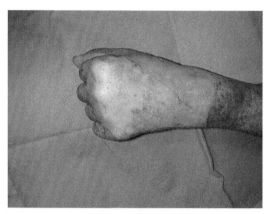

Fig. 15. Functional result at 3-month follow-up. (*Courtesy of* Eric Dantzer, MD, Toulon, France.)

inch thick. Wainwright[24] reported an 80% take rate in STSG less than 0.010 inch thick versus a 69% take rate for grafts greater than 0.010 inch thick. Additional advantages reported throughout the literature include increased elasticity, improved cosmesis, and improved functionality. Lattari and colleagues[25] found excellent functionality in terms of range of motion, grip strength, and fine motor coordination, in his case report on AlloDerm use in hands and feet, a study of only 3 cases. There were no reports of contracture formation in any of the case reports on AlloDerm use. On review of the literature on AlloDerm it is unclear why, despite these advantages, this dermal skin substitute is not more widely used today. Perhaps the problems with AlloDerm include the fact that it is highly sensitive to sheer forces, and that success of the grafts is highly dressing dependent[26] and dependent on the institution.[21]

Figs. 5–7 show the results of AlloDerm used for the reconstruction a hand following contracture release.

Integra

Integra (Integra Life Sciences, Plainsboro, New Jersey), an acellular collagen matrix composed of type I bovine collagen cross-linked with chondroitin-6-sulfate and covered by a thin silicone layer that serves as an epidermis,[27] was the first bioengineered skin approved by the FDA specifically designed to provide a neodermis to the wound bed. Integra has been approved for the initial coverage of excised acute burns and to treat severe burn scars.[28] The key to the successful use of Integra, as with any skin substitute, is its application on a meticulously excised wound that provides a cleaned, vascularized bed that is free from infection.

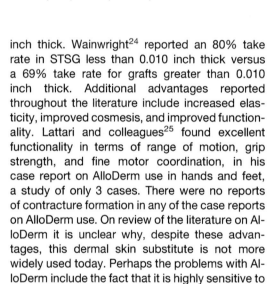

Fig. 14. Cosmetic result at 3-month follow-up. (*Courtesy of* Eric Dantzer, MD, Toulon, France.)

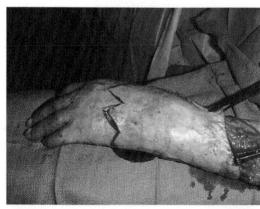

Fig. 16. Left hand of a 65-year-old woman; painful scar with limited range of motion 6 months post excision and grafting.

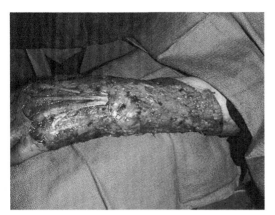

Fig. 17. Total scar excision including portions that encompassed the extensor tendons.

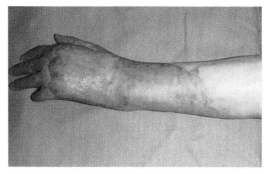

Fig. 19. Twelve months post thin epidermal graft to Integra.

The initial work with Integra in the treatment of large burns[29,30] was promising enough, after the initial learning curve, to tempt several surgeons to venture into the realm of using Integra for hand reconstruction following burn injury. Dantzer consistently achieved good functional and cosmetic outcomes for 33 cases in which Integra was used as a dermal matrix in both acute and reconstructive cases for hand burns. These studies also report 100% engraftment of the Integra and the initial STSG take was such that no additional grafts were needed for closure.[31,32]

Currently, Integra requires a 2-stage procedure. This 2-stage process is both an advantage and a disadvantage. Integra allows for an assured vascularized bed (Fig. 8), though one that must be nurtured to prevent silicone separation and watched closely for any sign of infection. The Vacuum Assisted Closure (V.A.C.) device (KCI, San Antonio, Texas) has been used to maintain contact between the silicone layer and the

collagen matrix of the Integra and perhaps to accelerate the vascularization of this bioengineered product.[33] The V.A.C. can be difficult to maintain and is usually changed twice weekly. If any pocket of fluid or infection is discovered, the areas should be sterilely drained through a small incision. The drainage should be sent for Gram stain, culture, and sensitivity. In the authors' hands, these dressing changes are performed with sterile techniques. Antibiotics are started according to prevalent cultures in the burn center at that time and adjusted according to culture results. Like Dantzer, the authors do not mesh Integra although many surgeons do.

Because the V.A.C. may be uncomfortable, needs to be changed 2 times a week, and does not allow the progress of the Integra to be tracked visually without changing the sponge, the authors are currently using TheraBond Antimicrobial Barrier (Choice Therapeutics, Natick, Massachsetts) to seal the seams and bolster the depressed areas. A Biobrane glove (UDL Laboratories Inc., Rockford, Illinois) is then used to provide enough pressure to keep the silicone attached to the underlying matrix

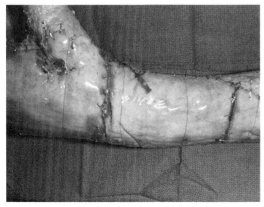

Fig. 18. Four weeks post scar excision and Integra application.

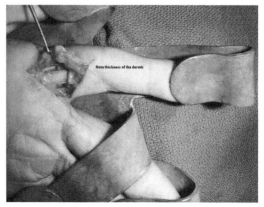

Fig. 20. Note thickness of "stacked Integra" layered neodermis at time of tenolysis.

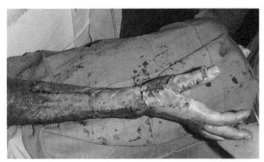

Fig. 21. Painful scars and limited range of motion 1 year post excision; skin graft required excision of scar and application of Integra. Intraoperative view before the application of a thin epidermal autograft.

(**Figs. 9** and **10**). This combination allows visualization of the Integra, does not require frequent dressing changes, and allows for gentle range of motion. Other centers have a different approach and mesh the Integra with a 1:1 noncrushing mesher (Brennen Medical-LLC, Saint Paul, Minnesota) and soak the matrix in Neosporin G.U. irrigant (Catalytica Pharmaceuticals Inc., Greenville, North Carolina), before application and then for cleaning the neodermis after the silicone layer has been removed. Quantitative cultures are also taken at the time of autografting and systemic antibiotics are started accordingly.[34]

Figs. **11–15** show the result of Integra used to treat an acute deep hand burn. The long-term follow-up shows an aesthetic result and full range of motion.

Integra has also been used in reconstruction for painful scars and contractures. **Figs. 16–18** demonstrate the use of Integra on the hand of a 65-year-old woman who sustained a full-thickness steam press

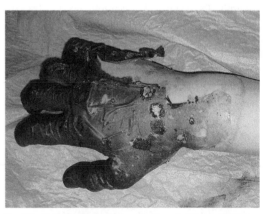

Fig. 23. Range of motion 1 year post Integra and thin epidermal graft.

injury. She was initially excised and grafted with a thick split-thickness skin graft within 72 hours of injury but, over a 3-month period, developed progressively limited range of motion and increased pain despite continued work with the occupational therapist. At the time of surgical exploration the scar was thick, and the initial excision at the junction of the graft and normal forearm skin released the tension and caused a large skin deficit (see **Fig. 16**). On excision of the remaining scar, it was seen that the hypertrophic scar actually encased portions of the extensor tendons (see **Fig. 17**). Due to the patient's family commitments, her second stage was delayed until 4 weeks after the Integra application. The Integra was an almond color (see **Fig. 18**) and had excellent petichial blood flow

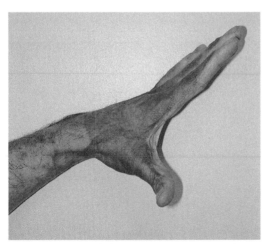

Fig. 22. One year follow-up post Integra and thin epidermal graft.

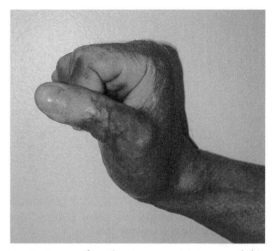

Fig. 24. Full-thickness burn to the right hand. (*From* Haslik W, Kamolz LP, Nathschlager G, et al. First experience with the collagen-elastin matrix Matriderm as a dermal substitute in severe burn injuries of the hand. Burns 2007;33(3):364–8; with permission.)

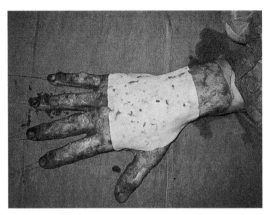

Fig. 25. Early, deep excision and immediate grafting with Matriderm. (*From* Haslik W, Kamolz LP, Nathschlager G, et al. First experience with the collagen-elastin matrix Matriderm as a dermal substitute in severe burn injuries of the hand. Burns 2007;33(3):364–8; with permission.)

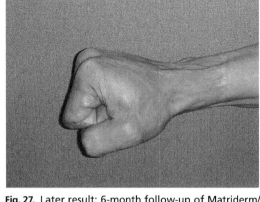

Fig. 27. Later result: 6-month follow-up of Matriderm/thin graft. (*From* Haslik W, Kamolz LP, Nathschlager G, et al. First experience with the collagen-elastin matrix Matriderm as a dermal substitute in severe burn injuries of the hand. Burns 2007;33(3):364–8; with permission.)

on dermabrasion. The thin epidermal graft (0.008 inch [0.020 cm]) had 100% engraftment. She had a marked reduction in pain and regained a functional range of motion, limited only by her preexisting arthritis (**Fig. 19**). Her pain was that she associated with her preexisting condition and was controlled with her usual anti-inflammatory agents.

Integra can also be stacked to correct soft tissue defects (**Fig. 20**). An electrical injury resulted in a defect at the base of the second metacarpophalangeal joint in addition to multiple other injuries in a 46-year-old man. The area was excised and covered by one layer of Integra without the silicone and then by one with the

silicone. Due to the stacking and concerns with vascularity following the electrical injury, the epithelial grafting was delayed for 6 weeks. The patient experienced a 100% take of the Integra and subsequent thin graft, but he developed an extension contracture due to adhesions, not to the neodermis, but to native tissue. At the time of tenolysis the thickness of the overlying dermis can be seen (see **Fig. 20**). He regained full range of motion following tenolysis and subsequent outpatient therapy.

Other examples of Integra used in reconstructive case are shown in **Figs. 21–23**. Although

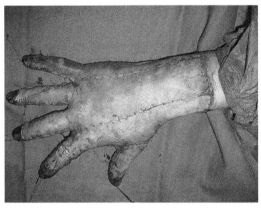

Fig. 26. Coverage of Matriderm with unmeshed skin grafts; V.A.C. or splint used for 5 days. (*From* Haslik W, Kamolz LP, Nathschlager G, et al. First experience with the collagen-elastin matrix Matriderm as a dermal substitute in severe burn injuries of the hand. Burns 2007;33(3):364–8; with permission.)

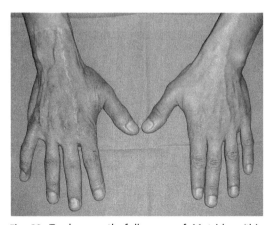

Fig. 28. Twelve-month follow-up of Matriderm/thin graft: right hand compared with noninjured left hand. (*From* Haslik W, Kamolz LP, Nathschlager G, et al. First experience with the collagen-elastin matrix Matriderm as a dermal substitute in severe burn injuries of the hand. Burns 2007;33(3):364–8; with permission.)

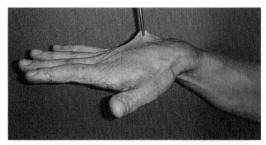

Fig. 29. Pliability of Matriderm/thin graft at 12-month follow-up. (*From* Haslik W, Kamolz LP, Nathschlager G, et al. First experience with the collagen-elastin matrix Matriderm as a dermal substitute in severe burn injuries of the hand. Burns 2007;33(3):364–8; with permission.)

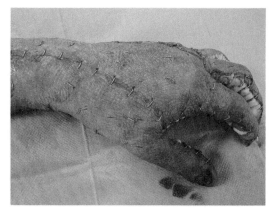

Fig. 31. Postoperative day 4, Matriderm/thin epidermal graft. (*Courtesy of* Eric Dantzer, MD, Toulon, France.)

Integra provides excellent soft tissue coverage, the timing of initiation of range of motion is still a concern and is limited not only by the rate of vascularization of the matrix but also by the experience of the occupational therapist and the type of dressing used. It seems that the Biobrane glove has provided an alternative to the V.A.C., allowing for better visualization and earlier range of motion. Care must be taken not to disrupt the attachment of the silicone to the matrix.

Although attempts to use Integra (without the silicone layer) as a single-stage reconstruction with immediate epidermal grafting have been attempted, the results to date are not of a quality for these authors to recommend. On the other hand, when used as a two-stage procedure on a clean wound bed, the authors agree with Dantzer and Braye[31] that Integra is an "alternative to full-thickness skin grafting, skin expansion, and even flaps for reconstructive surgery."

Although Integra is the most common permanent dermal regeneration template used in the

United States and now the standard to which the authors compare bioengineered dermal regenerative templates, it is not a panacea.[35] Integra is technique-specific, has a learning curve, requires a two-stage procedure, must be observed for infection, and is expensive. Therefore, the search for the ideal skin substitute continues.

Matriderm

Matriderm (Dr Oto Suwelack Skin and Health Care AG, Billerbeck, Germany) is a 1-mm thick dermal matrix composed of bovine dermis coated with elastin. The structurally intact type I, III, and V collagen is a three-dimensional structure coated with noncrossed linked elastin obtained from bovine nuchal ligaments.[36] The bioengineered skin substitute is used as a 1-step process with a thin autograft. Matriderm is currently not available in the United States but is widely used in Europe.

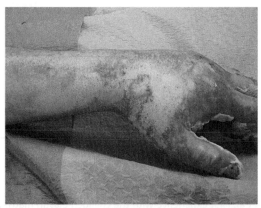

Fig. 30. Deep burn to the left forearm and hand of a 35-year-old man. (*Courtesy of* Eric Dantzer, MD, Toulon, France.)

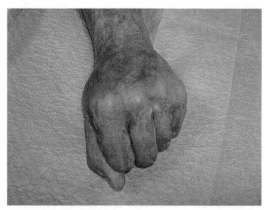

Fig. 32. Five-month functional result with Matriderm/thin epidermal graft. (*Courtesy of* Eric Dantzer, MD, Toulon, France.)

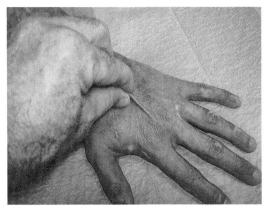

Fig. 33. Pliability of Matriderm/thin epidermal graft at 5-month follow-up. (*Courtesy of* Eric Dantzer, MD, Toulon, France.)

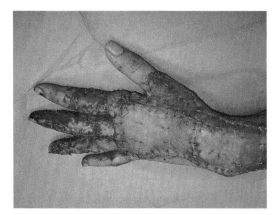

Fig. 35. Postoperative fascial excision and Matriderm/thin epidermal autograft. (*Courtesy of* Eric Dantzer, MD, Toulon, France.)

Promising results have been shown for hand reconstruction following thermal injuries in both the acute and reconstructive phases. The first clinical reports were published from the Medical University of Vienna in 2007.[36] The investigators felt the product should be considered because it involves a single-stage procedure and did not diminish the take of the autograft (95%), the patients achieved full range of motion, and the graft had good pliability. In a subsequent article in press, Haslik and colleagues[37] report the long-term results with sheet grafts over Matriderm in 17 patients. They obtained 96% take, no limitation in function, excellent cosmetic results, and pliability. In 5 patients in whom the size of the original defect could be accurately delineated, with no adjoining grafts or wounds that were allowed to heal without Matriderm/autograft, planimetry was performed. At 1 year follow-up, there was a modest 11% decrease in the size of the original wound.

Examples of the use of Matriderm for hand burns are shown in **Figs. 24–29**.

Dantzer has also had experience with Matriderm and is courteous enough to provide two of his cases for inclusion and comparison with the two-step technique of Integra (**Figs. 30–36**).

The early studies of Matriderm were not with hand burns and the results do not parallel those in hands. Van Zuijlen and colleagues[38] reported 73.4% graft take in acute burns versus 82.5% take without the skin substitute, a statistically significant difference. On the other hand, they showed no difference in reconstructive cases. Although this is much less than that reported for hand burns, the results of the initial study with Integra showed 80% initial matrix take.[29] Their reconstructive cases showed a 50% increase in pliability and a 33% increase in elasticity in the Matriderm cases. Long-term prospective studies including comparison with other dermal templates

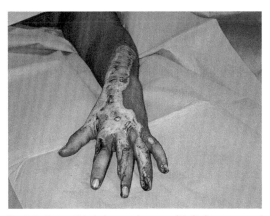

Fig. 34. Deep third-degree burns of left forearm and dorsal part of the hand of a 24-year-old woman. (*Courtesy of* Eric Dantzer, MD, Toulon, France.)

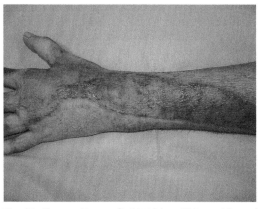

Fig. 36. Composite graft Matriderm/thin epidermal graft at 2-month follow-up. (*Courtesy of* Eric Dantzer, MD, Toulon, France.)

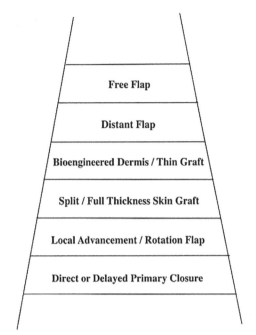

Fig. 37. Reconstructive ladder with additional consideration of bioengineered dermis and a thin epidermal autograft.

will be needed, but the potential for use in the United States is encouraging. A reliable, one-stage procedure for both acute and reconstructive cases would be welcome.

SUMMARY

In attempting to address the numerous bioengineered skin substitutes used for hand injuries, the surgeon must understand that the choice of an appropriate agent should be assessed on a case-by-case basis. This article presents a group of these agents either currently or soon to be available in the United States for temporary and permanent coverage. The authors do not attempt to cover all skin substitutes but rather those most commonly used for hand coverage. Some of these are clearly more pertinent and preferable in the senior author's experience and patient population. For temporary coverage, Biobrane and allograft have been the most commonly used skin substitutes. For permanent dermal regeneration, the authors have achieved the best results with Integra application followed by a staged placement of a thin epidermal autograft for use in the reconstruction of the hand. The senior author's results, though unpublished, show more than a 95% take rate with this technique. However, in reviewing the available agents, each has its own advantages and disadvantages in terms of functionality and aesthetics.

These factors should be weighed in the proper context along with the surgeon's clinical experience to maximize the chance for a superior outcome for both the patient and surgeon. This course of action obviously requires not only extensive communication with those more experienced with a particular agent but also an understanding that the best results may come after considering the learning curve involved. Oscar Wilde[39] once said "experience is simply the name we give our mistakes." If this is true, then persistence through early experience should lead the clinician to either adopt the use of the agent in his or her armamentarium or investigate other products. Again, it should be noted that no bioengineered skin product has fulfilled all the criteria for the ideal skin substitute by duplicating the complex structure and function of human skin. Some of the newer bioengineered products, including Matriderm, are currently unavailable in the United States but are in available in Europe. Once these are approved for use here, a more formal comparison of agents in a larger clinical trial would aid in determining how these products stand up to the current standard of care. The success of the bioengineered skin substitutes has allowed us to change our reconstructive ladder (**Fig. 37**), which now differs from the standard ladder taught in residency training programs.[40] It will be interesting to see in the near future which groundbreaking, revolutionary products in this rapidly expanding field will raise the standard to the next level.

REFERENCES

1. Luce EA. The acute and subacute management of the burned hand. Editor Luce, EA. Clin Plast Surg 2000;27(1):49–63.
2. Sheridan RL, Hurley J, Smith MA, et al. The acutely burned hand: management and outcome based on a ten-year experience with 1047 acute hand burns. J Trauma 1995;38(3):406–11.
3. Pereira C, Gold W, Herndon D. Review paper: burn coverage technologies: current concepts and future directions. J Biomater Appl 2007;22(2):101–21.
4. Porcine xenograft. Brennen medical. Available at: http://brennenmed.com/porcine.html. Accessed March 11, 2009.
5. Still J, Donker K, Law, et al. A program to decrease hospital stay in acute burn patients. Burns 1997; 23(6):498–500.
6. Hosseini SN, Mousavinasab SN, Fallahnezhat M. Xenoderm dressing in the treatment of second-degree burns. Burns 2007;33(6):776–81.
7. Smith DJ Jr. Use of Biobrane in wound management. J Burn Care Rehabil 1995;16(33):317–20.

8. Bishop JF, Demling RH, Hansbrough JF, et al. Biobrane summary. J Burn Care Rehabil 1995;16(33):341–2.

9. Lal S, Barrow RE, Wolf SE, et al. Biobrane improves wound healing in burned children without increased risk of infection. Shock 2000;14(3):314–8.

10. Whitaker IS, Worthington S, Jivan S, et al. The use of Biobrane by burn units in the United Kingdom: a national study. Burns 2007;33(8):1015–20.

11. Demling RH. Use of Biobrane in management of scalds. J Burn Care Rehabil 1995;16(3):329–30.

12. 510(k)s final decisions rendered for February 2009. U.S. Food and Drug Administration. Available at: http://www.fda.gov/cdrh/510k/sumfeb09.html; 2009. Accessed March 11, 2009.

13. Woodroof EA. The search for an ideal temporary skin substitute: AWBAT. Eplasty 2009;9:95–104.

14. Kagen RJ, Robb EC, Plessinger RT. The skin bank. In: Herndon DN, editor. Total burn care. 3rd edition. Philadelphia: Elsevier Health Sciences; 2007. p. 229–38.

15. May SR, DeClement SA. Development of a metabolic activity testing method for human and porcine skin. Cryobiology 1982;19(4):362–71.

16. Robb EC, Bechmann N, Plessinger RT, et al. A comparison of changed vs. unchanged media for viability testing of banked allograft skin. Presented at the 21th annual meeting of the American Association of Tissue Banks. San Diego (CA), August, 1997.

17. Cuono C, Langdon R, McGuire J. Use of cultured epidermal autografts and dermal allografts as skin replacement after burn injury. Lancet 1986;1(8490):1123–4.

18. Hickerson WL, Compton CC, Fletchall S, et al. Cultured epidermal autografts and allodermis combination for permanent burn wound coverage. Burns 1994;20(Suppl 1):1123–4.

19. Medawar PB. A second study of the behavior and fate of skin homografts in rabbits. J Anat 1945;79:157–76.

20. AlloDerm defined. LifeCell 2009. Available at: http://lifecell.com/products/95. Accessed March 11, 2009.

21. Wainwright D, Madden M, Lutterman A, et al. Clinical evaluation of an acellular allograft dermal matrix in full-thickness burns. J Burn Care Rehabil 1996;17(2):124–36.

22. Callcut RA, Schurr MJ, Sloan M, et al. Clinical experience with Alloderm: a one-staged composite dermal/epidermal replacement utilizing processed cadaver dermis and thin autografts. Burns 2006;32(5):583–8.

23. Bhavsar D, Tenehous M. The use of acellular dermal matrix for coverage of exposed joint and extensor mechanism in thermally injured patients with few options. Eplasty 2008;8:1–7.

24. Wainwright DJ. Use of an acellular allograft dermal matrix (Alloderm) in the management of full-thickness burns. Burns 1995;21(4):243–8.

25. Lattari V, Jones LM, Varcelott JR, et al. The use of a permanent dermal allograft in full thickness burns of the hand and foot: a report of three cases. J Burn Care Rehabil 1997;18(2):147–55.

26. Atiyeh BS, Hayek SN, Gunn SW. New technologies for burn wound closure and healing-review of the literature. Burns 2005;31(8):944–56.

27. Burke JF, Yannas IV, Quinby WL, et al. Successful use of a physiologically acceptable artificial skin in the treatment of extensive burn injury. Ann Surg 1981;194(4):413–28.

28. Integra dermal regeneration template. Food and Drug Administration 2002. Available at: http://www.fda.gov/cdrh/pdf/p900033s008.html. Accessed March 11, 2009.

29. Heinbach D, Luterman A, Burke J, et al. Artificial dermis for major burns: a multi-center randomized clinical trial. Ann Surg 1988;208(3):313–20.

30. Heinbach DM, Warden GD, Luterman A, et al. Multi-center postapproval clinical trial of Integra dermal regeneration template for burn treatment. J Burn Care Rehabil 2003;24(1):42–8.

31. Dantzer E, Braye FM. Reconstructive surgery using an artificial dermis (Integra): results with 39 grafts. Br J Plast Surg 2001;54(8):659–64.

32. Dantzer E, Queruel P, Salinier L, et al. Dermal regeneration template for deep hand burns: clinical utility for both early grafting and reconstructive surgery. Br J Plast Surg 2003;6(8):764–74.

33. Molnar JA, Defranzo AJ, Hadaegh A, et al. Acceleration of Integra incorporation in complex tissue defects with subatmospheric pressure. Plast Reconstr Surg 2004;113(5):1339–46.

34. Muangman P, Deubner H, Honari S, et al. Correlation of clinical outcome of Integra application with microbiologic and pathologic biopsies. J Trauma 2006;61(5):1212–7.

35. Jeng JC, Fidler PE, Sokolich JC, et al. Seven years experience with Integra as a reconstructive tool. J Burn Care Res 2007;28(1):120–6.

36. Haslik W, Kamolz LP, Nathschlager G, et al. First experience with the collagen-elastin matrix Matriderm as a dermal substitute in severe burn injuries of the hand. Burns 2007;33(3):364–8.

37. Haslik W, Kamolz LP, Manna F, et al. Management of full-thickness skin defects in the hand and wrist region: first long-term experiences with the dermal matrix Matriderm. J Plast Reconstr Aesthet Surg 2008;. doi:10.1016/j.bjps.2008.09.026.

38. van Zuijlen P, van Trier AJ, Vloemans JF, et al. Graft survival and effectiveness of dermal substitute in burns and reconstructive surgery in a one-stage grafting model. Plast Reconstr Surg 2000;106(3):615–23.

39. Wilde O. Lady Windermere's fan. In: The importance of being Ernest and other plays. London:1940.

40. Jensen AR, Klein MB, Halen JP, et al. Skin flaps and grafts: a primer for the national technical skills curriculum advanced tissue-handling module. J Surg Educ 2008;65(3):191–9.

Scar and Contracture: Biological Principles

Peter Kwan, MD[a], Keijiro Hori, MD[a], Jie Ding, PhD[a],
Edward E. Tredget, MD, MSc, FRCSC[a,b],*

KEYWORDS

- Burns • Contracture • Cicatrix • Hypertrophic scar
- Wound healing

SCOPE OF THE PROBLEM

As the primary interface between humans and their environment, the hands are constantly exposed to danger. As a result, burn injuries of the hand are common. In toddlers these are often scald burns that occur during exploration of the environment,[1] whereas in adults these are often flame or flash burns resulting from occupational or recreational injuries.[2,3] In both these groups the potential for lifelong morbidity resulting from loss of function is enormous. According to the Centers for Disease Control (CDC) more than 400,000 nonfatal burn injuries occurred in the United States of America in 2007.[4] Of these, 45% involved the arm and hand.[5] The resulting potential for significant functional impairment and hypertrophic scarring (HTS) is high,[6] making a hand burn one of the American Burn Association (ABA) criteria for mandatory referral to a burn center.[7]

Whereas many of these hand burns are superficial and often heal without sequelae, deeper burns are prone to increased scarring and contracture,[8–10] as shown in **Fig. 1**. Those hand injuries that lead to poor scar are also prone to scar contracture. It is often this secondary contracture that leads to the greatest functional impairment (**Fig. 2**). As the primary means of interaction with the physical environment, function and appearance of the hand are crucial.[11,12] Scarring and contracture both lead to impaired hand function.[13] Understanding the underlying biologic mechanisms involved allows the hand surgeon to better address these issues, and suggests new avenues of research to improve patient outcome.[14]

The stages of normal wound healing have been well described by several investigators.[15–19] In this article, the authors review the underlying biology of scar and contracture by focusing on potential causes of abnormal wound healing, and explore therapeutic measures designed to target the various biologic causes of poor scar.

PATHOPHYSIOLOGY OF SCAR
Injury Beyond a Critical Depth Leads to Scar Formation Rather than Regeneration

Although determination of the depth of injury is beyond the scope of this article, it is well known that the difference between superficial and deep burns is of great clinical importance and largely determines how these injuries heal and the degree of scarring to be expected.[9,10] Superficial wounds traditionally are those expected to heal within 2 weeks without surgical intervention.[10] Deep wounds are prone to HTS and contracture[20] and surgical intervention, including the application of split thickness skin grafts, is typically used in an attempt to avoid these sequelae.[21] On the other hand, superficial wounds usually heal with a minimum of scarring[20] and are generally

This work was supported by the Firefighters' Burn Trust Fund of the University of Alberta Hospital and the Canadian Institutes of Heath Research.
[a] Division of Plastic and Reconstructive Surgery, Department of Surgery, 2D2.28 WMC, University of Alberta, 8440-112 Street, Edmonton, AB T6G 2B7, Canada
[b] Division of Critical Care, Department of Surgery, 2D2.28 WMC, University of Alberta, 8440-112 Street, Edmonton, AB T6G 2B7, Canada
* Corresponding author.
E-mail address: etredget@ualberta.ca (E.E. Tredget).

Hand Clin 25 (2009) 511–528
doi:10.1016/j.hcl.2009.06.007
0749-0712/09/$ – see front matter © 2009 Published by Elsevier Inc.

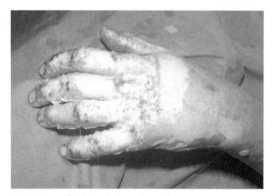

Fig. 1. Superficial and deep hand burns.

managed with dressings to facilitate the body's natural reparative mechanisms.[22] These clinical observations correlate with the wound healing seen in an experimental dermal scratch model developed by Dunkin and colleagues.[23] In this model, a jig was used to create a linear skin wound that increased in depth along its length from no injury to full-thickness injury.[23] The investigators observed that superficial injury less than 0.56 mm in depth (or 33.1% of normal hip skin thickness) resulted in regeneration rather than scar whereas deeper injury resulted in increasing scar formation.[23] This result suggests that injury beyond a critical depth leads to scar formation rather than regeneration (Fig. 3). The reasons for this are currently unclear; however, two major hypotheses have been proposed: (1) selective proliferation of fibroblast subpopulations resulting from fibrogenic cytokines, and (2) thermal injury destroying a subpopulation of fibroblasts thus leaving a distinct phenotype of deeper fibroblasts to repopulate the wound.[24] Indeed, several studies have shown that superficial and deep fibroblasts respond differently to injury.[25–33] This difference, to be discussed further, may be one of the keys

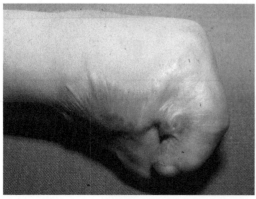

Fig. 2. Scar contractures in a hand burn.

to understanding HTS formation following burn injury.[24] Thus not only does depth of injury play a crucial role in dictating clinical management but it also suggests new aspects of the pathophysiology of wound healing to be explored.

Fibrogenic and Antifibrogenic Cytokines Modulate Fibroblasts

The local cellular environment exerts great control over the healing process. Local cytokines serve as the signaling molecules that modulate the activity of fibroblasts and keratinocytes, causing them to close and heal wounds or become overactive, leading to HTS.[34] The balance between profibrotic and antifibrotic cytokines (Fig. 4) has a great impact on the eventual wound-healing outcome.

Platelet-derived growth factor (PDGF) is produced in wound healing by platelets from the injured capillaries. Four subtypes have been described, which form dimers to activate two structurally related tyrosine kinase receptors.[35] Activation causes cellular proliferation and actin reorganization, making PDGF a potent mitogen on mesenchymal cells (MSC) including fibroblasts, and induces their transformation into myofibroblasts.[36] PDGF increases extracellular matrix (ECM) production and inhibits myofibroblast apoptosis.[37] PDGF has been implicated in scleroderma, pulmonary fibrosis, hepatic fibrosis, and various renal diseases.[38] Dermal fibroblasts not only respond to PDGF but produce it as well, resulting in an autocrine loop, and PDGF also increases transforming growth factor-β (TGF-β) receptors in scleroderma fibroblasts.[39] The effect of PDGF is increased in HTS and keloid fibroblasts,[40] all suggesting that PDGF may play a role in fibrosis and abnormal scarring of skin. Thus it may be further suggested that blocking PDGF via tyrosine kinase inhibitors could reduce fibrosis and improve clinical outcomes, which it does in several murine models of radiation-induced pulmonary fibrosis[41] and scleroderma.[42]

TGF-β is the prototypic profibrotic cytokine and belongs to a large superfamily of cytokines sharing a conserved cysteine knot structure.[43,44] When initially produced it is usually bound to an associated latent TGF-β binding protein (LTBP) in an inactive form. This bond is cleaved, to activate TGF-β, by several enzymes present in blood or released during cell injury, including matrix metalloproteinase-2 (MMP-2), MMP-9, and plasmin.[45] Three known isoforms exist in mammals: β1, β2, and β3,[44] and are produced by a multitude of sources including degranulating platelets, macrophages, T lymphocytes, endothelial cells, keratinocytes, and fibroblasts.[46] TGF-β1/2 acts

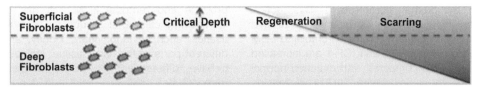

Fig. 3. Regeneration occurs in superficial wounds while scarring occurs in deeper wounds.

via the Smad pathway to regulate several cellular processes related to fibrosis.[47] TGF-β acts as a chemoattractant for monocytes[48] and fibroblasts,[49] stimulates fibroblasts to produce ECM,[50] and modulates production of several proteinases and their inhibitors.[51] TGF-β is upregulated locally in tissue and systemically in serum in burn patients with HTS,[52] and fibroblasts from HTS synthesize greater amounts of TGF-β than normal dermal fibroblasts.[53] Fetal wounds, which normally regenerate rather than form scar, can be induced to form scar tissue by exposure to TGF-β1.[54] Taken together, these results suggest TGF-β seems to be a key initiator of fibrosis and HTS. Although most isoforms of TGF-β are profibrotic, several studies have shown improved wound healing when exposed to TGF-β3.[55,56] TGF-β3 is strongly induced in the later stages of wound healing and reduces ECM deposition,[57] which may be one factor in its mechanism of action.

Connective tissue growth factor (CTGF) is one of the original members of the CCN protein family.[58] CTGF is a downstream regulator of fibrosis that is induced by TGF-β[59,60] and upregulates ECM production by fibroblasts.[61] It seems that CTGF and TGF-β independently induce only transient fibrosis, whereas when combined they lead to prolonged fibrosis.[62] CTGF is upregulated in scleroderma, HTS,[63] and many other fibrotic conditions.[64] In these chronic conditions fibrosis continues due to CTGF, even though TGF-β becomes downregulated.[60] This fact suggests that although TGF-β is important in initiating pathologic scarring, it is CTGF that sustains the fibrotic process. CTGF seems to be induced by TGF-β via the ras/MEK/ERK pathway, and blocking this pathway using iloprost reduces fibrosis[65] as does anti-CTGF antibody or CTGF siRNA.[66]

Insulin like growth factor-1 (IGF-1) modulates growth hormone effects on various tissues including dermal fibroblasts.[67] IGF-1 is a fibroblast[68] and endothelial cell[69] mitogen and induces collagen production in osteoblasts,[70] human pulmonary fibroblasts,[71] and human dermal fibroblasts.[72] IGF-1 is expressed locally in injured tissue and this parallels granulation tissue formation up to 5 weeks post injury.[73] Not only does IGF-1 stimulate glycosaminoglycan and collagen production, but it also reduces collagenase mRNA levels and

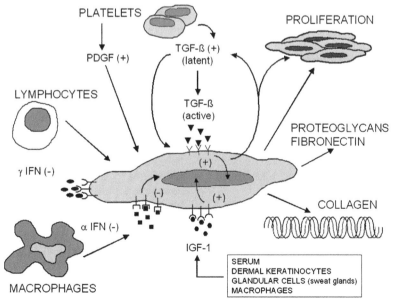

Fig. 4. Balance of profibrotic and antifibrotic factors in wound healing. (*From* Scott PG, Ghahary A, Tredget EE. Molecular and cellular aspects of fibrosis following thermal injury. Hand Clin 2000;16(2):271–87; with permission.)

activity by dermal fibroblasts.[74] This action adversely impacts the critical balance of collagen production and degradation that is crucial to ECM remodeling. Both TGF-β and IGF-1 are increased in postburn HTS compared with matched normal dermis from the same patients,[75] in a similar fashion to other fibrotic conditions including scleroderma, pulmonary fibrosis, and hepatic fibrosis.[24] It has been shown that in skin, IGF-1 is restricted to epidermal sweat and sebaceous glands where dermal fibroblasts are not exposed to it.[24,75] In wounds such as burns, where these structures are damaged, dermal fibroblasts would be exposed to IGF-1 and this could contribute to HTS formation. Once the epidermal wound has healed this exposure would cease and could account for the observation that wounds reepithelializing within 2 weeks are less prone to HTS than those taking longer to heal and expose fibroblasts to IGF-1 for extended periods of time.[24] In addition, IGF-1 has been shown to act as a TGF-β stimulating factor.[72] Although IGF-1 may not be the only cause of fibrotic growth factor in HTS, these findings suggest it has an important role in concert with TGF-β in the pathogenesis of abnormal scarring.

HTS is not simply due to the presence of fibrogenic cytokines alone, as many are present in both normal scar and HTS, albeit in differing quantities. Likely just as important is the relative decrease in several antifibrotic cytokines and the delicate balance between the two. Two antifibrotic cytokines of great interest are interferon-α2b (IFN-α2b) and IFN-γ. IFN-α is produced by leukocytes and fibroblasts whereas IFN-γ is produced by Th1 T helper cells,[76] all of which are known to play a role in wound healing. IFNs decrease ECM production by dermal fibroblasts from fibroproliferative lesions to normal levels.[24] IFN-α2b also increases dermal fibroblast collagenase expression and decreases tissue inhibitor of matrix metalloproteinase (TIMP-1).[77] A prospective clinical trial by the authors' research group in postburn patients showed reductions in HTS volume, normalized TGF-β levels, and reduced scar angiogenesis after treatment with subcutaneous IFN-α2b.[52] This result suggests that in the treatment of abnormal scar and contracture, increasing antifibrotic cytokines is just as important as reducing profibrotic ones.

Dermal Fibroblast Subpopulations Including Myofibroblasts Behave Differently in Wound Healing

Fibroblasts are one of the key players in wound healing, and serve as the primary MSC of scar formation and contraction. Fibroblasts participate in the physical aspects of wound closure and also produce and remodel ECM.[15] It has become increasingly clear that fibroblasts from different tissues, such as lung, heart, kidney, and even different parts of the same tissue, including skin, behave differently.[32,78] Recent studies have demonstrated that superficial and deep dermal fibroblasts, derived from the papillary and reticular layers, behave differently. Compared with superficial fibroblasts, deeper fibroblasts produce more collagen,[25] proliferate more slowly,[26,27] produce greater contraction of collagen gels,[29] produce less decorin,[30] induce more irregular keratinocyte proliferation,[31] and are not as supportive of the formation of capillaries by vascular endothelial cells.[33] This heterogeneity of fibroblasts may account for the different patterns of healing seen with varying depths of injury.

It has been proposed that when superficial fibroblasts are destroyed by deep thermal injuries the deeper fibroblasts remain to repopulate and heal the wound, contributing to HTS formation.[24] In a mouse model in which human skin was grafted onto animals and subsequently injured, deep dermal fibroblasts were found to initially close the experimental wounds, which were then remodeled by superficial fibroblasts.[79] It is possible that insufficient numbers of superficial fibroblasts to remodel the ECM contributes to HTS formation. HTS fibroblasts certainly appear similar in behavior to deep dermal fibroblasts as compared with superficial fibroblasts, when their production and response to cytokines as well as production of ECM is examined.[80] Studies conducted in the authors' laboratory show that TGF-β and CTGF, two key profibrotic cytokines, are produced in greater quantities by deeper fibroblasts,[80] which mirrors their increased production demonstrated in HTS fibroblasts.[53,63] This result suggests that the biology of HTS fibroblasts is directly related to that of deep dermal fibroblasts, and that models and therapeutic measures targeted at deep dermal fibroblasts, which are simpler to obtain and more easily studied, will provide insight into HTS.

Myofibroblasts are a particular phenotype of fibroblasts, initially described by Majno and colleagues,[81] and are widely associated with contraction.[82] Myofibroblasts differ from fibroblasts by their expression of α-smooth muscle actin (α-SMA)[83] and several other aspects of their behavior. Myofibroblasts produce more collagen and less collagenase than fibroblasts[84] and are more numerous in HTS than normal scar.[85,86] HTS myofibroblasts are less sensitive to apoptotic signals and this, coupled with their increased production of ECM, may be a direct factor in HTS formation.[87]

Fibrocytes are a Systemic Source of Fibroblasts and Myofibroblasts and also Regulators of Preexisting Wound-Healing Cells

Fibrocytes are a leukocyte subpopulation similar to monocytes, but express collagen and participate in the regulation of fibroblasts and wound healing.[88] Fibrocytes were first described by Bucala and colleagues[88] in 1994, who observed a blood-borne cell that behaved like a fibroblast in wound chambers implanted on the backs of mice. Fibrocytes are uniquely identified by double staining for procollagen I, and CD34[88] or leukocyte specific protein-1 (LSP-1).[89] Since their initial description, fibrocytes have been found in normal healing[90] and in several fibroproliferative diseases including pulmonary fibrosis,[91,92] nephrogenic fibrosis,[93] atherosclerotic lesions,[94] chronic pancreatitis,[95] and chronic cystitis,[96] as well as hypertrophic burn scars.[97–99] Abe and colleagues[90] showed that secondary lymphoid chemokine (SLC), a C-C chemokine ligand of CCR7, promotes fibrocyte migration to wounds and is produced by the vascular endothelium in wounds, suggesting SLC plays a role in fibrocyte trafficking to wounds. It has been shown that fibrocytes are upregulated in burn patients[97] and they are hypothesized to contribute to abnormal scarring through several different mechanisms.[100] When exposed to profibrotic cytokines, fibrocytes produce large amounts of ECM and differentiate into myofibroblasts via activation of the Smad2/3 and SAPK/JNK MAPK pathways.[101] Pilling and colleagues[102] identified serum amyloid P (SAP), a constitutive plasma protein related to C-reactive protein (CRP), as an inhibitor of fibrocyte differentiation from CD14+ peripheral blood monocytes. These investigators showed that sera from patients with scleroderma low in SAP does not inhibit fibrocyte differentiation[102] and, in a murine bleomycin model of pulmonary fibrosis, used SAP injections to inhibit fibrocyte differentiation and reduce collagen production, fibrocytes, and leukocytes in the lung.[103]

Fibrocytes may be more than simply another source of fibroblasts and myofibroblasts in healing wounds. Fibrocytes may be a crucial link between the immune system and healing wounds and serve as regulators of preexisting wound-healing fibroblasts and other cells. Fibrocytes, true to their leukocyte lineage, are capable of acting as antigen-presenting cells (APC) and can prime naïve T cells.[104] Fibrocytes also express Toll-like receptors (TLR) on their cell surfaces, allowing them to respond as part of the innate immune system to a large variety of invading pathogens.[105] Furthermore, a study by Wang and colleagues[89] in burn patients suggests that fibrocytes regulate the activity of preexisting fibroblasts by producing TGF-β and CTGF (**Fig. 5**). Fibrocytes may also play an important role in revascularization of healing wounds by secreting MMP-9, which degrades matrix and promotes endothelial cell invasion while

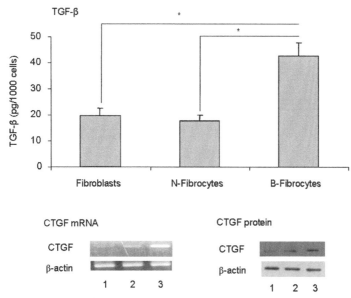

Fig. 5. TGF-β and CTGF production by fibrocytes in normal and burn patients. (*From* Wang J, Jiao H, Stewart TL, et al. Fibrocytes from burn patients regulate the activities of fibroblasts. Wound Repair Regen 2007;15(1):113–21; with permission.)

also producing several proangiogenic factors including vascular endothelial growth factor (VEGF).[106]

Keratinocytes Interact with Fibroblasts to Control Wound Healing

Keratinocytes play a crucial role in wound healing, with reepithelialization serving as a key end point in scar formation. Wounds taking longer than 2 weeks to reepithelialize are at increased risk of HTS.[107] This fact suggests that keratinocytes interact with fibroblasts to control scarring.[108,109] Keratinocytes do regulate the action of fibroblasts and vice versa.[110,111] Keratinocytes suppress TGF-β and CTGF production by fibroblasts.[112] Keratinocyte coculture and keratinocyte-conditioned media modulate fibroblasts by increasing proliferation but simultaneously decrease ECM synthesis, in part, via keratinocyte-derived antifibrogenic factor (KDAF), subsequently identified as stratifin (14-3-3 Sigma).[113] This action may occur via increased MMP-1 production from KDAF-stimulated fibroblasts.[113] In contrast, several investigators have demonstrated that keratinocytes from HTS induce cocultured fibroblasts to produce increased ECM compared with keratinocytes from normal skin.[114] This result suggests that abnormal regulation of keratinocyte-fibroblast crosstalk may be an important component of HTS formation.

Immune System and T Lymphocytes Regulate Wound Healing

Clinical observation suggests that injuries leading to a prolonged immune response seem to increase the risk of fibroproliferative scar. However, recent research suggests that the type of immune response rather than degree of inflammation is the predisposing factor.[115] Mast cells, neutrophils, and macrophages all play a role in the initial inflammatory state of wound healing.[116] Macrophages, in particular, are involved in the transition from inflammation to proliferation. Macrophages produce proinflammatory cytokines including interleukin-1 (IL-1), IL-6, and tumor necrosis factor-α (TNF-α), which control inflammatory cell adhesion and migration, and also stimulate keratinocytes and fibroblasts to proliferate.[36] Macrophages also produce known profibrogenic factors including PDGF, TGF-β, and IGF-1.[117] In a CXCR3 knockout mouse model, it was shown that CXCR3 is a key receptor used by macrophages to infiltrate healing wounds, and that its inactivation leads to reduced wound healing.[118] This result suggests that macrophages are a key component of the transition from inflammation to proliferation, and could also play a role in the initial stages of HTS formation.

T-helper cells (CD4+) seem to act as immunoregulators that produce various cytokines to control the wound-healing process (**Fig. 6**).[100] In burn injury, once activated by macrophages,[119] dendritic cells,[120] or APC, naïve T-helper cells become polarized toward a Th1 or Th2 type[121] and produce specific cytokine profiles.[122] Samples of HTS dermis demonstrated increased CD4+ T lymphocyte infiltration compared with normal skin in the same patients.[123] Although Th1 cells are classically considered the primary actors in cell-mediated immunity, they also

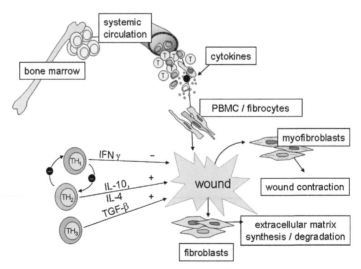

Fig. 6. Hypothetical diagram of the role of Th1/Th2/Th3 cells in stimulating bone marrow stem cells to healing wounds. (*From* Armour J, Scott PG, Tredget EE. Cellular and molecular pathology of HTS: basis for treatment. Wound Repair Regen 2007;15:S6–17; with permission.)

produce mainly antifibrotic cytokines (IL-2, IFN-γ, and IL-12), induce fibroblast proapoptotic genes, and activate nitric oxide synthase (NOS) expression, which promotes collagenase activity.[124] In contrast, whereas Th2 cells are classically associated with antibody-mediated immunity, they also produce primarily profibrotic cytokines including IL-4, which has twice the profibrotic potency of TGF-β in fibroblasts, IL-5, and IL-13. Th2-linked genes upregulate ECM production and include procollagens I, III, and V, arginase-1, MMP-2, MMP-9, and tissue inhibitor of TIMP-1.[125] In burn patients, serum samples show elevated Th2 cytokine levels of IL-4 and IL-10, and reduced Th1 cytokine levels of IFN-γ and IL-12 for over 1 year post injury.[126,127] Cultured fibroblasts treated with serum from burn patients resulted in Th2 polarized responses including increased cellular proliferation, TGF-β upregulation, and expression of α-SMA, suggesting a transformation to the myofibroblast phenotype.[123]

Extracellular Matrix Influences Cellular Behavior

The ECM formed during initial wound closure is ultimately remodeled as wound healing and scar formation occur. A complex interplay exists between fibroblasts and the ECM environment with which they interact.[82,128] ECM conceptually has two major components: collagen fibrils that are responsible for tensile strength, and glycosaminoglycans that contribute to tissue osmotic pressure and provide resistance to compression.[24] Clinically HTS is raised, erythematous, and firm to the touch.[129] In structural terms HTS ECM contains dense nodules of poorly organized, thin collagen fibrils in whorl-like patterns, which appear encapsulated in more normal-appearing collagen. In contrast, normal dermis contains thick parallel collagen bundles and fibers.[130,131] ECM formed in HTS is thicker, is hyperhydrated, and has overlying epidermis that is also often thicker.[24] This disorganization may be due in part to alterations in the collagen fibers and proteoglycans present in HTS compared with normal tissue.

Although the dry weight of HTS collagen is reduced in comparison with normal dermis or mature scar, because of its increased thickness HTS does have more collagen per unit surface area.[24] Abnormal collagen fibrils may be due in part to alterations in the relative proportions of the various collagen types. Although normal dermis and scar are predominantly 80% type I, 10% to 15% type III, and minimal type V, the ratios in HTS are very different with ~33% type III and up to 10% type V.[132–134] Both type III and type V

collagen have been shown to alter the fibril diameter of type I collagen bundles, and the different ratios in HTS may account for some morphologic changes in ECM structure.[135–137]

The relative content of several glycosaminoglycans is also altered in HTS.[138] Overall, there is more than a two-fold increase in glycosaminoglycans, leading to greater hydration and likely causing the increased clinical firmness of HTS.[24] Proteoglycans also influence collagen fibril morphology, cell-matrix interactions, and cellular behavior. The most plentiful proteoglycan in normal dermis is decorin, which is reduced by 75% in HTS.[138] This finding is significant in that decorin has been shown to have a multitude of roles including modulation of collagen fibrils,[139,140] regulation of TGF-β,[141,142] and reduction of fibrosis[143,144] and contraction.[145,146] Two other proteoglycans, versican and biglycan, are upregulated in HTS to compensate for the lack of decorin. In particular, versican is increased 6-fold above the normal level and from its position between collagen fibrils may contribute to increased tissue turgor and an expanded collagen network of ECM, leading to the increased scar volume seen in HTS.[24]

PATHOPHYSIOLOGY OF CONTRACTURE

When discussing contracture a key distinction must be drawn between the wound contracture that occurs as a part of the initial closure and healing process, and the scar contracture that occurs as the scar matures. Wound contraction is the biologic means whereby the edges of an open wound are pulled together by forces resulting from the wound-healing process. In contrast, scar contraction is the shrinkage that occurs in an already healed scar.[84,147]

Although most contraction research continues to occur in animal models, wound contraction plays a greater role in wound healing in animals as compared with humans.[148,149] Scar contractures result from HTS over joints and mobile surfaces that contract secondarily, but HTS only occurs in humans,[84] making discovery of a good in vivo experimental animal model crucial to further research.[150] Wound contraction is usually assessed by photographic analysis of standardized wounds created on the backs of animals. Alternatively, in vitro contraction models consist of fibroblast-populated collagen lattices (FPCL) whereby collagen is solubilized, seeded with fibroblasts, and polymerized at 37°C before measurement of the change in surface area or diameter of the lattice over time.[151]

It is generally accepted that the fibroblast and myofibroblast are involved in wound and scar contraction, although the relative roles of each vary depending on the theory. Two theories on the mechanism of contraction have been proposed: (1) myofibroblasts and (2) fibroblast locomotion and shape changes.[84] The first theory involves myofibroblasts, a specialized type of fibroblast, which produce α-SMA and possess thick cytoplasmic stress fibers.[82] It has been hypothesized that wound contraction involves cell shortening via α-SMA that then rearrangement of the surrounding connective tissue due to cell-to-cell contact.[152] It seems that myofibroblasts contribute to the excessive ECM present in HTS. This excess ECM probably contributes to the rigidity of HTS and reduces movement, leading to scar contracture.[84,153] The second theory suggests that fibroblasts cause contraction by exerting a traction force as they propel themselves through connective tissue with filipodia.[154,155] This theory is supported by the delayed predominance of myofibroblasts in healing wounds until a week after the majority of wound contraction has already occurred.[84] It has been suggested that myofibroblasts function not to cause contraction but rather to maintain a static equilibrium that already exists within tissue.[156] This function is consistent with experiments demonstrating that tension applied to skin[157] and scar[86] caused the appearance of myofibroblasts, suggesting myofibroblasts may not play a large role in wound contracture but may instead be primarily responsible for scar contracture.

Wound Contraction is Primarily Caused by Fibroblasts

Wound contraction is affected by the same variety of factors as scar formation. In FPCL the rate of contraction is accelerated by increased fibroblast density or decreased collagen concentration.[158] The cytoskeleton is another key factor in contraction of FPCL, and presumably healing wounds. Although fibroblasts in FPCL are initially spherical they subsequently form a bipolar configuration,[159,160] following rearrangement of their microfilaments, considered necessary for contraction.[161,162] When FPCL are examined shortly after contraction begins there appear to be two cell subpopulations present. Fibroblasts with numerous cytoplasmic microfilaments, characteristic of myofibroblasts, are localized to the edges whereas bipolar fibroblasts are predominant at the center.[84] When the relative contractile abilities of these subpopulations are compared the bipolar fibroblasts are far more

contractile, again suggesting that fibroblasts instead of myofibroblasts are the major cell responsible for wound contraction.[156,163] As well, the environmental cytokines have a significant effect on the contractile process. TGF-β increases the rate and degree of contraction without upregulating proliferation,[164,165] and it has been postulated that this may be through the induction of PDGF.[166] In contrast, IFN-α2b reduced contraction of FPCL by fibroblasts, possibly by downregulating cytoplasmic actin filaments[167] or increasing apoptosis.[168] In the FPCL model the type of collagen also has a significant effect on contraction rates. Lattices with increased type III collagen,[169] similar to HTS, display increased contraction rates, as do lattices of collagen taken from HTS.[156] Increased decorin expression by transfection inhibited FPCL contraction.[145] Decorin normally modulates collagen fibril formation[139,140] and neutralizes TGF-β.[141,142] Thus, in HTS, where decorin is significantly reduced, these factors may also add to wound contraction. The influence of ECM on wound contraction is further reinforced by the observation that contraction does not occur in frostbite injuries in which cells are necrotic but ECM remains intact.[170]

Scar Contraction is Primarily Caused by Myofibroblasts

Scar contraction is still a poorly understood process. Well-known clinical risk factors include HTS.[76] The most predominant theories involve myofibroblasts.[84] It is well known that primary split thickness skin grafting is more effective in inhibiting wound contraction than delayed grafting,[171] and more rapid scar maturation in animal models is associated with a more rapid reduction in myofibroblast population[172] secondary to the induction of apoptosis.[173,174] Using fibroblasts and myofibroblasts isolated from HTS resulted in myofibroblasts playing a greater role in scar contracture.[175] This result suggests that myofibroblasts are the primary cell involved in scar contracture whereas fibroblasts are the primary cell involved in wound contracture. TGF-β is upregulated in HTS and increases the contractile forces of HTS fibroblasts, leading to scar contracture.[176] Scar contractures clinically appear most frequently over joints and mobile surfaces.[84] In burn wounds, HTS tensile forces induce transdifferentiation of fibroblasts into myofibroblasts.[86] Mechanical stress has also been shown to downregulate proapoptotic genes in fibroblasts.[177] This result helps explain the predominance of myofibroblasts in scar contractures and why they do not undergo apoptosis as in a regular scar, and suggests that modulation of myofibroblast behavior is likely key to reducing scar contracture.

PATHOPHYSIOLOGY OF TREATMENTS
Nonsurgical Treatment

Pressure garments
Pressure garments have been the major treatment modality for HTS since the early 1970s.[178] The garments must be worn continuously for at least 23 hours a day and must be applied until the scar is mature, which can take 2 or 3 years.[179] The exact pressure required for effective treatment has never been scientifically established but most investigators believe that pressures should exceed capillary pressure and recommend that pressure be maintained between 24 and 30 mm Hg.[180] It is thought that pressure may accelerate scar maturation and reduce the incidence of contractures. Also, pressure garments may help to alleviate the itchiness and pain associated with active HTS. A systematic meta-analysis of the evidence for use of pressure garment therapy revealed that there was a small, but statistically significant improvement in scar height. However, there was no significant difference for the outcomes of scar pigmentation, vascularity, pliability, and color.[181] In terms of pathophysiology, pressure garments control collagen synthesis, reduce collagen production, and encourage realignment of collagen bundles already present.[179] Although the exact mechanism of pressure garment therapy for the treatment of HTS is not fully understood, some of the possible mechanisms are increased myofibroblast apoptosis, a decrease in collagen synthesis, ischemic cell damage, and an increase in MMP-9 activity.[115]

Silicone gel sheets
Silicone gel sheeting has been used for treatment of immature burn scars since it was introduced by Perkins and colleagues in 1982.[182] Silicone gel, which is the cross-linked polymer of dimethylsiloxane, needs to be in place for at least 12 hours a day for 3 to 6 months.[183] Silicone gel sheets may accelerate scar maturation and improve pigmentation, vascularity, pliability, and itchiness associated with HTS.[184] Although the mechanism of silicone-based products in the treatment of HTS management has not been completely determined, some of the mechanisms of action suggested include an increase of skin temperature, development of a static electrical field, increased stratum corneum hydration, decreased TGF-β2 levels, increased fibroblast apoptosis, decreased mast cell numbers, and a decrease in fibroblast-mediated contraction.[115]

Splinting
Patients with severe hand burns are subject to joint contractures that can lead to claw hand deformities (**Fig. 2**). This intrinsic-minus position of the hand is due to increased fluid accumulation in the joints capsule, swelling of the collateral ligaments by fluid imbibition, and subsequent ligament contraction.[185] To avoid the contracture, optimal positioning of the hand is important.[186] Splints should be applied in intrinsic-plus position in which the wrist is slightly extended to 20° to 30°, the metacarpophalangeal (MCP) joint flexed with approximately 80°, interphalangeal (IP) joints are completely extended, and the thumb is placed in maximum abduction. Splinting is sufficient at night, and active and passive exercises with the hand should be performed twice a day. Range of motion should be avoided in patients with deep dermal or full-thickness burns, where there is suspicion of an imminent injury to the extensor tendon apparatus to prevent rupture of the tendons.[185]

Immunologic and Biomolecular Therapies

Corticosteroids
Intralesional corticosteroid injections have been used for the treatment of pathologic scars since the mid-1960s[187] and remain the first line of treatment. Triamcinolone acetonide is the most commonly used concentration, with injection of 10 to 40 mg/mL at 2- to 6-week intervals.[180,188,189] Injection should be confined to the papillary dermis to avoid subcutaneous atrophy.[189] The mechanisms involved are complex and remain unclear. However, it is understood that corticosteroids inhibit the proliferation and contraction of fibroblasts, suppress inflammation by inhibition of leukocyte and monocyte migration and phagocytosis, increase hypoxia by vasoconstriction, increase collagenase production by inhibition of α2-macroglobulin, and inhibit growth factors such as TGF-β and IGF-1.[115,189,190]

5-Fluorouracil
5-Fluorouracil (5-FU) is a pyramidine analogue with antimetabolite activity, which is one of the antimitotic agents and is used as a chemotherapy drug. 5-FU has also been used for glaucoma-filtering surgery,[191] the treatment of basal cell carcinoma and keratoacanthoma,[192] and treatment of keloids and HTS.[193,194] Intralesional injection of 5-FU (50 mg/mL) alone or in combination with corticosteroids and pulsed-dye laser decrease the size, and soften and flatten the abnormal scar.[192–195] 5-FU targets rapidly proliferating fibroblasts in dermal wounds, which leads to

inhibition of fibroblast proliferation and a decrease in fibroblast collagen production.[196]

Interferon

The IFN family is an antifibrotic cytokine that consists of type 1 IFN (including IFN-α and IFN-β) and type 2 IFN (IFN-γ). The IFNs are capable of decreasing the excessive production of collagen and glycosaminoglycans by scar-forming fibroblasts and normalizing the subnormal level of collagenase activity.[197] IFN-α and IFN-γ have antagonized TGF-β protein production.[198] IFN-α decreases cell proliferation, collagen, fibronectin synthesis, and fibroblast-mediated wound contracture,[76,167] which relates to a decrease of TGF-β and mast cell histamine production. IFN-α also reduces the collagenase inhibitor TIMP-1.[77] IFN-γ increases myofibroblast apoptosis[199] and inhibits collagen synthesis but decreases collagenase activity.[77,200] Subcutaneous IFN-α2b injection significantly improved scar quality and volume, and sustained reduced serum TGF-β levels even after treatment.[52] However, intralesional interferon injections have not been found to be effective in scar modulation.[201]

Transforming growth factor-β

TGF-β has been implicated in wound healing and HTS.[180] There are 3 mammalian isoforms of TGF-β (TGF-β1, TGF-β2, and TGF-β3). TGF-β1 and TGF-β2 have been identified as promoters of collagen synthesis and scarring, whereas TGF-β3 has been linked with scar prevention.[189,190] Several studies have targeted TGF-β effects by reducing Smad-3 and increasing Smad-7 with neutralizing antibodies. Natural inhibitors of TGF-β, which do not block wound healing and the immune system, such as LTBP-1, latency-associated protein (LAP), decorin, and biglycan, have been also studied for inhibition of TGF-β mediated biologic effects.[115,189] Mannose 6-phosphate (M6P) has been injected into wounds to inhibit proteolytic activation of TGF-β from its latent form.[202,203] In a rat cutaneous wound model, Shah and colleagues[204] demonstrated significant reduction of scarring with exogenous addition of neutralizing antibody of TGF-β1 and TGF-β2 or exogenous addition of recombinant TGF-β3. Further investigation of TGF-β3 injection to the wound demonstrated an improvement of ECM deposition.[55] In recent studies recombinant human TGF-3 intradermal injection, 50 to 500 ng/100 μL/linear cm wound margin around the time of surgery, showed significant improvement in scar appearance.[205,206]

Surgical Treatment

Scar revision surgery

HTS resulting from excessive tension or delay of wound closure can be treated effectively with surgery. There are many surgical options that include intramarginal excision, skin grafts, local flaps, and free flaps, although the surgical method used will depend on the extent and region of the scar and contracture, as well as the size of the tissue defect after the abnormal scar has been excised. In general, these techniques are not appropriate for immature hypertrophic scar.[180]

Laser therapies

Laser therapies were introduced for HTS by Apfelberg and colleagues and Castro and colleagues in the mid-1980s. There are 2 major kinds of lasers: ablative nonselective lasers such as CO_2 laser and erbium:YAG laser, and nonablative selective lasers such as pulsed-dye laser and Nd:YAG laser. CO_2 laser and erbium:YAG laser have a high affinity for water. These lasers cause thermal necrosis, which promotes wound contraction and collagen remodeling.[207] Pulsed-dye lasers are effective in the improvement of scar texture, redness, size, and pliability.[208,209] The mechanism of this laser therapy is based on selective photothermolysis, in which the light energy emitted from a vascular laser is absorbed by oxyhemoglobin, generating heat and leading to coagulation necrosis.[210] Kuo and colleagues found suppression of fibroblast proliferation and collagen type III deposition and downregulation of TGF-β1 expression correlated with upregulation of MMP-13 (collagenase-3) activity.[210]

Cryosurgery

Shepherd and Dawber were the first to apply cryosurgery as a monotherapy regimen for treating HTS and keloids in1982. Cryosurgery required up to 20 treatment sessions with 2 to 3 spray or contact freeze-thaw cycles of 15 to 30 seconds each.[189] Cryosurgery reduces the volume and helps to soften the lesions but the side effect of permanent hypopigmentation is a major handicap.[190] However, recently an intralesional needle cryoprobe method has been developed to improve the efficacy and avoid the side effects.[211] The mechanism of cryosurgery is based on the low temperatures, which cause blood stasis, cell anoxia, and necrosis, leading to increase of fibroblast apoptosis and decrease of vascularity.[115,189]

Stem cells and tissue engineering

Early excision of burn tissue and early wound closure improve HTS and joint contracture.[212] Because of the limited use of donor site, dermal substitutes have been developed. Autologous and allogeneic skin substitutes are composed of keratinocytes or fibroblasts, in part combined with allogenic (fibrin) or xenogeneic (collagen, hyaluronan) matrix substances.[213] Cultured epithelial autograft was used from 1981 onward for the treatment of full-thickness burn[214] but it was fragile and the graft take rate was relatively low without the dermal component. The noncellular components of the dermis, which primarily consist of ECM proteins and collagen,[215] have been developed and attempts have been made to improve the rapid vascularization of dermal substitutes whereby growth factors such as VEGF and fibroblast growth factor (FGF) have been used to accelerate vascularization, but with modest benefit.[216] In a mouse model, Kataoka and colleagues[217] demonstrated the potential of bone marrow-derived cells (BMDCs) to be differentiated into cells composing the skin such as epidermal keratinocytes, sebaceous gland cells, follicular epithelial cells, dendritic cells, and endothelial cells. In another study, bone marrow-derived mesenchymal stem cells (BM-MSCs) accelerated cutaneous wound healing, which is thought to be contributed by the transdifferentiation of human BM-MSCs into the epithelium.[218]

SUMMARY

Fibroproliferative disorders underlie a wide variety of human diseases spanning most major organ systems. In hand burns, HTS continues to be a major source of morbidity. Increased understanding of the basic biology and pathophysiology of abnormal scarring, as reviewed here, is providing new and exciting avenues of research and potential clinical therapeutics for a difficult problem. It is to be hoped that advances in fibroproliferative research will ultimately provide better outcomes for those with hand burns and a multitude of other diseases.

REFERENCES

1. Ewings EL, Pollack J. Pediatric upper extremity burns: outcomes of emergency department triage and outpatient management. J Burn Care Res 2008;29(1):77–81.
2. Islam SS, Nambiar AM, Doyle EJ, et al. Epidemiology of work-related burn injuries: experience of a state-managed workers' compensation system. J Trauma 2000;49(6):1045–51.
3. Fagenholz PJ, Sheridan RL, Harris NS, et al. National study of emergency department visits for burn injuries, 1993 to 2004. J Burn Care Res 2007;28(5):681–90.
4. Centers for Disease Control. WISQARS: nonfatal injury reports. Atlanta (GA): Centers for Disease Control; 2008.
5. Pruitt BA, Wolf SE, Mason AD, et al. Epidemiological, demographic and outcome characteristics of burn injury. In: Herndon DN, editor. Total burn care. Philadelphia: Saunders; 2007. p. 14–32.
6. Bombaro KM, Engrav LH, Carrougher GJ, et al. What is the prevalence of hypertrophic scarring following burns? Burns 2003;29(4):299–302.
7. American Burn Association. Guidelines for the operation of burn centers. J Burn Care Res 2007; 28(1):134–41.
8. van Zuijlen PP, Kreis RW, Vloemans AF, et al. The prognostic factors regarding long-term functional outcome of full-thickness hand burns. Burns 1999; 25(8):709–14.
9. Gangemi EN, Gregori D, Berchialla P, et al. Epidemiology and risk factors for pathologic scarring after burn wounds. Arch Facial Plast Surg 2008; 10(2):93–102.
10. Monstrey S, Hoeksema H, Verbelen J, et al. Assessment of burn depth and burn wound healing potential. Burns 2008;34(6):761–9.
11. Robson MC, Smith DJ, VanderZee AJ, et al. Making the burned hand functional. Clin Plast Surg 1992; 19(3):663–71.
12. Greenhalgh DG, Vu HL. Acute management of the burned hand and electrical injuries. In: Mathes SJ, editor. Plastic surgery. Philadelphia: Saunders; 2006. p. 587–603.
13. Bayat A, McGrouther DA, Ferguson MWJ. Skin scarring. BMJ 2003;326(7380):88–92.
14. Engrav LH, Garner WL, Tredget EE. Hypertrophic scar, wound contraction and hyper-hypopigmentation. J Burn Care Res 2007;28(4):593–7.
15. Singer AJ, Clark RAF. Cutaneous wound healing. N Engl J Med 1999;341(10):738–46.
16. Rhett J, Ghatnekar G, Palatinus J, et al. Novel therapies for scar reduction and regenerative healing of skin wounds. Trends Biotechnol 2008;26(4): 173–80.
17. Martin P. Wound healing—aiming for perfect skin regeneration. Science 1997;276(5309):75–81.
18. Clark RAF, Ghosh K, Tonnesen MG. Tissue engineering for cutaneous wounds. J Invest Dermatol 2007;127(5):1018–29.
19. Baum CL, Arpey CJ. Normal cutaneous wound healing: clinical correlation with cellular and molecular events. Dermatol Surg 2005;31(6):674–86 [discussion: 686].
20. Cubison TCS, Pape SA, Parkhouse N. Evidence for the link between healing time and the development of hypertrophic scars (HTS) in paediatric burns due to scald injury. Burns 2006;32(8):992–9.

21. Engrav LH, Heimbach DM, Reus JL, et al. Early excision and grafting vs. nonoperative treatment of burns of indeterminant depth: a randomized prospective study. J Trauma 1983;23(11): 1001–4.

22. Wasiak J, Cleland H, Campbell F. Dressings for superficial and partial thickness burns. Cochrane Database Syst Rev 2008;(4):CD002106.

23. Dunkin CSJ, Pleat JM, Gillespie PH, et al. Scarring occurs at a critical depth of skin injury: precise measurement in a graduated dermal scratch in human volunteers. Plast Reconstr Surg 2007; 119(6):1722–32.

24. Scott PG, Ghahary A, Tredget EE. Molecular and cellular aspects of fibrosis following thermal injury. Hand Clin 2000;16(2):271–87.

25. Ali-Bahar M, Bauer B, Tredget EE, et al. Dermal fibroblasts from different layers of human skin are heterogeneous in expression of collagenase and types I and III procollagen mRNA. Wound Repair Regen 2004;12(2):175–82.

26. Feldman SR, Trojanowska M, Smith EA, et al. Differential responses of human papillary and reticular fibroblasts to growth factors. Am J Med Sci 1993; 305(4):203–7.

27. Harper RA, Grove G. Human skin fibroblasts derived from papillary and reticular dermis: differences in growth potential in vitro. Science 1979; 204(4392):526–7.

28. Lochner K, Gaemlich A, Sudel KM, et al. Expression of decorin and collagens I and III in different layers of human skin in vivo: a laser capture microdissection study. Biogerontology 2007;8(3): 269–82.

29. Schafer IA, Shapiro A, Kovach M, et al. The interaction of human papillary and reticular fibroblasts and human keratinocytes in the contraction of three-dimensional floating collagen lattices. Exp Cell Res 1989;183(1):112–25.

30. Schonherr E, Beavan LA, Hausser H, et al. Differences in decorin expression by papillary and reticular fibroblasts in vivo and in vitro. Biochem J 1993; 290(Pt 3):893–9.

31. Sorrell JM, Baber MA, Caplan AI. Site-matched papillary and reticular human dermal fibroblasts differ in their release of specific growth factors/cytokines and in their interaction with keratinocytes. J Cell Physiol 2004;200(1):134–45.

32. Sorrell JM, Caplan AI. Fibroblast heterogeneity: more than skin deep. J Cell Sci 2004;117(Pt 5): 667–75.

33. Sorrell JM, Baber MA, Caplan AI. Human dermal fibroblast subpopulations; differential interactions with vascular endothelial cells in coculture: nonsoluble factors in the extracellular matrix influence interactions. Wound Repair Regen 2008;16(2): 300–9.

34. Barrientos S, Stojadinovic O, Golinko MS, et al. Growth factors and cytokines in wound healing. Wound Repair Regen 2008;16(5):585–601.

35. Andrae J, Gallini R, Betsholtz C. Role of platelet-derived growth factors in physiology and medicine. Genes Dev 2008;22(10):1276–312.

36. Werner S, Grose R. Regulation of wound healing by growth factors and cytokines. Physiol Rev 2003; 83(3):835–70.

37. Powell DW, Mifflin RC, Valentich JD, et al. Myofibroblasts. I. Paracrine cells important in health and disease. Am J Phys 1999;277(1 Pt 1):C1–9.

38. Bonner JC. Regulation of PDGF and its receptors in fibrotic diseases. Cytokine Growth Factor Rev 2004;15(4):255–73.

39. Trojanowska M. Role of PDGF in fibrotic diseases and systemic sclerosis. Rheumatology (Oxford) 2008;47(Suppl 5):v2–4.

40. Younai S, Venters G, Vu S, et al. Role of growth factors in scar contraction: an in vitro analysis. Ann Plast Surg 1996;36(5):495–501.

41. Abdollahi A, Li M, Ping G, et al. Inhibition of platelet-derived growth factor signaling attenuates pulmonary fibrosis. J Exp Med 2005;201(6):925–35.

42. Distler JHW, Jungel A, Huber LC, et al. Imatinib mesylate reduces production of extracellular matrix and prevents development of experimental dermal fibrosis. Arthritis Rheum 2007;56(1):311–22.

43. Gordon K, Blobe G. Role of transforming growth factor-β superfamily signaling pathways in human disease. Biochim Biophys Acta 2008;1782(4): 197–228.

44. Prud'homme GJ. Pathobiology of transforming growth factor b in cancer, fibrosis and immunologic disease, and therapeutic considerations. Lab Invest 2007;87(11):1077–91.

45. Leask A, Abraham DJ. TGF-beta signaling and the fibrotic response. FASEB J 2004;18(7):816–27.

46. Roberts AB. Molecular and cell biology of TGF-beta. Miner Electrolyte Metab 1998;24(2–3): 111–9.

47. Cutroneo KR. TGF-beta-induced fibrosis and SMAD signaling: oligo decoys as natural therapeutics for inhibition of tissue fibrosis and scarring. Wound Repair Regen 2007;15(Suppl 1):S54–60.

48. Wakefield LM, Smith DM, Masui T, et al. Distribution and modulation of the cellular receptor for transforming growth factor-beta. J Cell Biol 1987; 105(2):965–75.

49. Postlethwaite AE, Keski-Oja J, Moses HL, et al. Stimulation of the chemotactic migration of human fibroblasts by transforming growth factor beta. J Exp Med 1987;165(1):251–6.

50. Ignotz RA, Massague J. Transforming growth factor-beta stimulates the expression of fibronectin and collagen and their incorporation into the extracellular matrix. J Biol Chem 1986;261(9):4337–45.

51. Edwards DR, Murphy G, Reynolds JJ, et al. Transforming growth factor beta modulates the expression of collagenase and metalloproteinase inhibitor. EMBO J 1987;6(7):1899–904.

52. Tredget EE, Shankowsky HA, Pannu R, et al. Transforming growth factor-beta in thermally injured patients with hypertrophic scars: effects of interferon alpha-2b. Plast Reconstr Surg 1998;102(5): 1317–28 [discussion: 1329–30].

53. Wang R, Ghahary A, Shen Q, et al. Hypertrophic scar tissues and fibroblasts produce more transforming growth factor-beta1 mRNA and protein than normal skin and cells. Wound Repair Regen 2000;8(2):128–37.

54. Lanning DA, Nwomeh BC, Montante SJ, et al. TGF-beta1 alters the healing of cutaneous fetal excisional wounds. J Pediatr Surg 1999;34(5):695–700.

55. Occleston NL, Laverty HG, O'Kane S, et al. Prevention and reduction of scarring in the skin by transforming growth factor beta 3 (TGFbeta3): from laboratory discovery to clinical pharmaceutical. J Biomater Sci Polym Ed 2008;19(8):1047–63.

56. Occleston NL, O'Kane S, Goldspink N, et al. New therapeutics for the prevention and reduction of scarring. Drug Discov Today 2008;13(21–22):973–81.

57. Bock O, Yu H, Zitron S, et al. Studies of transforming growth factors beta 1-3 and their receptors I and II in fibroblast of keloids and hypertrophic scars. Acta Derm Venereol 2005;85(3):216–20.

58. Perbal B. CCN proteins: multifunctional signalling regulators. Lancet 2004;363(9402):62–4.

59. Grotendorst GR. Connective tissue growth factor: a mediator of TGF-beta action on fibroblasts. Cytokine Growth Factor Rev 1997;8(3):171–9.

60. Leask A, Abraham DJ. The role of connective tissue growth factor, a multifunctional matricellular protein, in fibroblast biology. Biochem Cell Biol 2003;81(6):355–63.

61. Ihn H. Pathogenesis of fibrosis: role of TGF-beta and CTGF. Curr Opin Rheumatol 2002;14(6): 681–5.

62. Mori T, Kawara S, Shinozaki M, et al. Role and interaction of connective tissue growth factor with transforming growth factor-beta in persistent fibrosis: a mouse fibrosis model. J Cell Physiol 1999; 181(1):153–9.

63. Colwell AS, Phan T-T, Kong W, et al. Hypertrophic scar fibroblasts have increased connective tissue growth factor expression after transforming growth factor-beta stimulation. Plast Reconstr Surg 2005; 116(5):1387–90 [discussion: 1391–82].

64. Shi-Wen X, Leask A, Abraham D. Regulation and function of connective tissue growth factor/CCN2 in tissue repair, scarring and fibrosis. Cytokine Growth Factor Rev 2008;19(2):133–44.

65. Stratton R, Shiwen X, Martini G, et al. Iloprost suppresses connective tissue growth factor production in fibroblasts and in the skin of scleroderma patients. J Clin Invest 2001;108(2):241–50.

66. Abraham D. Connective tissue growth factor: growth factor, matricellular organizer, fibrotic biomarker or molecular target for anti-fibrotic therapy in SSc? Rheumatology (Oxford) 2008; 47(Suppl 5):v8–9.

67. Jones JI, Clemmons DR. Insulin-like growth factors and their binding proteins: biological actions. Endocr Rev 1995;16(1):3–34.

68. Rolfe KJ, Cambrey AD, Richardson J, et al. Dermal fibroblasts derived from fetal and postnatal humans exhibit distinct responses to insulin like growth factors. BMC Dev Biol 2007;7(124):1–13.

69. Miele C, Rochford JJ, Filippa N, et al. Insulin and insulin-like growth factor-I induce vascular endothelial growth factor mRNA expression via different signaling pathways. J Biol Chem 2000;275(28): 21695–702.

70. Hill DJ, Logan A, McGarry M, et al. Control of protein and matrix-molecule synthesis in isolated ovine fetal growth-plate chondrocytes by the interactions of basic fibroblast growth factor, insulin-like growth factors-I and -II, insulin and transforming growth factor-beta 1. J Endocrinol 1992;133(3):363–73.

71. Goldstein RH, Poliks CF, Pilch PF, et al. Stimulation of collagen formation by insulin and insulin-like growth factor I in cultures of human lung fibroblasts. Endocrinology 1989;124(2):964–70.

72. Ghahary A, Shen Q, Shen YJ, et al. Induction of transforming growth factor beta 1 by insulin-like growth factor-1 in dermal fibroblasts. J Cell Physiol 1998;174(3):301–9.

73. Steenfos HH, Jansson JO. Gene expression of insulin-like growth factor-I and IGF-I receptor during wound healing in rats. Eur J Surg 1992; 158(6–7):327–31.

74. Ghahary A, Shen YJ, Nedelec B, et al. Collagenase production is lower in post-burn hypertrophic scar fibroblasts than in normal fibroblasts and is reduced by insulin-like growth factor-1. J Invest Dermatol 1996;106(3):476–81.

75. Ghahary A, Shen YJ, Wang R, et al. Expression and localization of insulin-like growth factor-1 in normal and post-burn hypertrophic scar tissue in human. Mol Cell Biochem 1998;183(1–2):1–9.

76. Tredget EE, Nedelec B, Scott PG, et al. Hypertrophic scars, keloids, and contractures. The cellular and molecular basis for therapy. Surg Clin North Am 1997;77(3):701–30.

77. Ghahary A, Shen YJ, Nedelec B, et al. Interferons gamma and alpha-2b differentially regulate the expression of collagenase and tissue inhibitor of metalloproteinase-1 messenger RNA in human hypertrophic and normal dermal fibroblasts. Wound Repair Regen 1995;3(2):176–84.

78. Nolte SV, Xu W, Rennekampff H-O, et al. Diversity of fibroblasts—a review on implications for skin tissue engineering. Cells Tissues Organs 2008;187(3): 165–76.

79. Rossio-Pasquier P, Casanova D, Jomard A, et al. Wound healing of human skin transplanted onto the nude mouse after a superficial excisional injury: human dermal reconstruction is achieved in several steps by two different fibroblast subpopulations. Arch Dermatol Res 1999; 291(11):591–9.

80. Wang J, Dodd C, Shankowsky HA, et al. Deep dermal fibroblasts contribute to hypertrophic scarring. Lab Invest 2008;88(12):1278–90.

81. Majno G, Gabbiani G, Hirschel BJ, et al. Contraction of granulation tissue in vitro: similarity to smooth muscle. Science 1971;173(996):548–50.

82. Hinz B, Gabbiani G. Cell-matrix and cell-cell contacts of myofibroblasts: role in connective tissue remodeling. Thromb Haemost 2003;90(6): 993–1002.

83. Sappino AP, Schurch W, Gabbiani G. Differentiation repertoire of fibroblastic cells: expression of cytoskeletal proteins as marker of phenotypic modulations. Lab Invest 1990;63(2):144–61.

84. Nedelec B, Ghahary A, Scott PG, et al. Control of wound contraction. Basic and clinical features. Hand Clin 2000;16(2):289–302.

85. Ehrlich HP, Desmouliere A, Diegelmann RF, et al. Morphological and immunochemical differences between keloid and hypertrophic scar. Am J Pathol 1994;145(1):105–13.

86. Junker JPE, Kratz C, Tollback A, et al. Mechanical tension stimulates the transdifferentiation of fibroblasts into myofibroblasts in human burn scars. Burns 2008;34(7):942–6.

87. Moulin VR, Larochelle SB, Langlois CL, et al. Normal skin wound and hypertrophic scar myofibroblasts have differential responses to apoptotic inductors. J Cell Physiol 2004;198(3):350–8.

88. Bucala R, Spiegel LA, Chesney J, et al. Circulating fibrocytes define a new leukocyte subpopulation that mediates tissue repair. Mol Med 1994;1(1):71–81.

89. Wang JF, Jiao H, Stewart TL, et al. Fibrocytes from burn patients regulate the activities of fibroblasts. Wound Repair Regen 2007;15(1):113–21.

90. Abe R, Donnelly SC, Peng T, et al. Peripheral blood fibrocytes: differentiation pathway and migration to wound sites. J Immunol 2001; 166(12):7556–62.

91. Moeller A, Gilpin S, Ask K, et al. Circulating fibrocytes are an indicator for poor prognosis in idiopathic pulmonary fibrosis. Am J Respir Crit Care Med 2009;179(7):588–94.

92. Phillips RJ. Circulating fibrocytes traffic to the lungs in response to CXCL12 and mediate fibrosis. J Clin Invest 2004;114(3):438–46.

93. Bellini A, Mattoli S. The role of the fibrocyte, a bone marrow-derived mesenchymal progenitor, in reactive and reparative fibroses. Lab Invest 2007; 87(9):858–70.

94. Medbury HJ, Tarran SLS, Guiffre AK, et al. Monocytes contribute to the atherosclerotic cap by transformation into fibrocytes. Int Angiol 2008;27(2): 114–23.

95. Barth PJ, Ebrahimsade S, Hellinger A, et al. CD34+ fibrocytes in neoplastic and inflammatory pancreatic lesions. Virchows Arch 2002;440(2): 128–33.

96. Nimphius W, Moll R, Olbert P, et al. CD34+ fibrocytes in chronic cystitis and noninvasive and invasive urothelial carcinomas of the urinary bladder. Virchows Arch 2007;450(2):179–85.

97. Yang L, Scott PG, Giuffre J, et al. Peripheral blood fibrocytes from burn patients: identification and quantification of fibrocytes in adherent cells cultured from peripheral blood mononuclear cells. Lab Invest 2002;82(9):1183–92.

98. Yang L, Scott PG, Dodd C, et al. Identification of fibrocytes in postburn hypertrophic scar. Wound Repair Regen 2005;13(4):398–404.

99. Holland AJA, Tarran SLS, Medbury HJ, et al. Are fibrocytes present in pediatric burn wounds? J Burn Care Res 2008;29(4):619–26.

100. Wynn TA. Cellular and molecular mechanisms of fibrosis. J Pathol 2008;214(2):199–210.

101. Hong KM, Belperio JA, Keane MP, et al. Differentiation of human circulating fibrocytes as mediated by transforming growth factor-beta and peroxisome proliferator-activated receptor gamma. J Biol Chem 2007;282(31):22910–20.

102. Pilling D, Buckley CD, Salmon M, et al. Inhibition of fibrocyte differentiation by serum amyloid P. J Immunol 2003;171(10):5537–46.

103. Pilling D, Roife D, Wang M, et al. Reduction of bleomycin-induced pulmonary fibrosis by serum amyloid P. J Immunol 2007;179(6):4035–44.

104. Chesney J, Bacher M, Bender A, et al. The peripheral blood fibrocyte is a potent antigen-presenting cell capable of priming naive T cells in situ. Proc Natl Acad Sci U S A 1997;94(12):6307–12.

105. Balmelli C, Alves MP, Steiner E, et al. Responsiveness of fibrocytes to Toll-like receptor danger signals. Immunobiology 2007;212(9–10):693–9.

106. Hartlapp I, Abe R, Saeed RW, et al. Fibrocytes induce an anglogenic phenotype in cultured endothelial cells and promote angiogenesis in vivo. FASEB J 2001;15(12):2215–24.

107. Deitch EA, Wheelahan TM, Rose MP, et al. Hypertrophic burn scars: analysis of variables. J Trauma 1983;23(10):895–8.

108. Colwell AS, Yun R, Krummel TM, et al. Keratinocytes modulate fetal and postnatal fibroblast transforming growth factor-beta and Smad expression

in co-culture. Plast Reconstr Surg 2007;119(5): 1440–5.

109. Ghahary A, Ghaffari A. Role of keratinocyte-fibro-blast cross-talk in development of hypertrophic scar. Wound Repair Regen 2007;15(Suppl 1): S46–53.

110. Werner S, Krieg T, Smola H. Keratinocyte-fibroblast interactions in wound healing. J Invest Dermatol 2007;127(5):998–1008.

111. Ghaffari A, Kilani RT, Ghahary A. Keratinocyte-conditioned media regulate collagen expression in dermal fibroblasts. J Invest Dermatol 2009; 129(2):340–7.

112. Amjad SB, Carachi R, Edward M. Keratinocyte regulation of TGF-beta and connective tissue growth factor expression: a role in suppression of scar tissue formation. Wound Repair Regen 2007; 15(5):748–55.

113. Ghahary A, Marcoux Y, Karimi-Busheri F, et al. Differentiated keratinocyte-releasable stratifin (14-3-3 sigma) stimulates MMP-1 expression in dermal fibroblasts. J Invest Dermatol 2005;124(1):170–7.

114. Bellemare J, Roberge CJ, Bergeron D, et al. Epidermis promotes dermal fibrosis: role in the pathogenesis of hypertrophic scars. J Pathol 2005;206(1):1–8.

115. Armour A, Scott PG, Tredget EE. Cellular and molecular pathology of HTS: basis for treatment. Wound Repair Regen 2007;15(Suppl 1):S6–17.

116. van der Veer WM, Bloemen MCT, Ulrich MMW, et al. Potential cellular and molecular causes of hypertrophic scar formation. Burns 2009;35(1): 15–29.

117. Sunderkotter C, Steinbrink K, Goebeler M, et al. Macrophages and angiogenesis. J Leukoc Biol 1994;55(3):410–22.

118. Ishida Y, Gao J-L, Murphy PM. Chemokine receptor CX3CR1 mediates skin wound healing by promoting macrophage and fibroblast accumulation and function. J Immunol 2008;180(1): 569–79.

119. Goodman RE, Nestle F, Naidu YM, et al. Keratinocyte-derived T cell costimulation induces preferential production of IL-2 and IL-4 but not IFN-gamma. J Immunol 1994;152(11):5189–98.

120. Hauser C. The interaction between langerhans cells and CD4+ T cells. J Dermatol 1992;19(11): 722–5.

121. Romagnani S. Th1 and Th2 in human diseases. Clin Immunol Immunopathol 1996;80(3 Pt 1):225–35.

122. Mosmann TR, Coffman RL. Th1 and Th2 cells: different patterns of lymphokine secretion lead to different functional properties. Annu Rev Immunol 1989;7:145–73.

123. Wang J, Jiao H, Stewart TL, et al. Increased TGF-beta-producing CD4+ T lymphocytes in postburn patients and their potential interaction with dermal

fibroblasts in hypertrophic scarring. Wound Repair Regen 2007;15(4):530–9.

124. Wynn TA. Fibrotic disease and the T(H)1/T(H)2 paradigm. Nat Rev Immunol 2004;4(8):583–94.

125. Sandler NG, Mentink-Kane MM, Cheever AW, et al. Global gene expression profiles during acute pathogen-induced pulmonary inflammation reveal divergent roles for Th1 and Th2 responses in tissue repair. J Immunol 2003;171(7):3655–67.

126. Kilani RT, Delehanty M, Shankowsky HA, et al. Fluorescent-activated cell-sorting analysis of intracellular interferon-gamma and interleukin-4 in fresh and frozen human peripheral blood T-helper cells. Wound Repair Regen 2005;13(4):441–9.

127. Tredget EE, Yang L, Delehanty M, et al. Polarized Th2 cytokine production in patients with hypertrophic scar following thermal injury. J Interferon Cytokine Res 2006;26(3):179–89.

128. Wang H-J, Pieper J, Schotel R, et al. Stimulation of skin repair is dependent on fibroblast source and presence of extracellular matrix. Tissue Eng 2004; 10(7–8):1054–64.

129. Niessen FB, Spauwen PH, Schalkwijk J, et al. On the nature of hypertrophic scars and keloids: a review. Plast Reconstr Surg 1999;104(5): 1435–58.

130. Linares HA, Kischer CW, Dobrkovsky M, et al. The histiotypic organization of the hypertrophic scar in humans. J Invest Dermatol 1972;59(4): 323–31.

131. Kischer CW. Collagen and dermal patterns in the hypertrophic scar. Anat Rec 1974;179(1):137–45.

132. Hayakawa T, Hashimoto Y, Myokei Y, et al. Changes in type of collagen during the development of human post-burn hypertrophic scars. Clin Chim Acta 1979;93(1):119–25.

133. Bailey AJ, Bazin S, Sims TJ, et al. Characterization of the collagen of human hypertrophic and normal scars. Biochim Biophys Acta 1975;405(2):412–21.

134. Ehrlich HP, White BS. The identification of alpha A and alpha B collagen chains in hypertrophic scar. Exp Mol Pathol 1981;34(1):1–8.

135. Lapiere CM, Nusgens B, Pierard GE. Interaction between collagen type I and type III in conditioning bundles organization. Connect Tissue Res 1977; 5(1):21–9.

136. Adachi E, Hayashi T. In vitro formation of hybrid fibrils of type V collagen and type I collagen. Limited growth of type I collagen into thick fibrils by type V collagen. Connect Tissue Res 1986; 14(4):257–66.

137. Birk DE, Fitch JM, Babiarz JP, et al. Collagen fibrillogenesis in vitro: interaction of types I and V collagen regulates fibril diameter. J Cell Sci 1990; 95(Pt 4):649–57.

138. Scott PG, Dodd CM, Tredget EE, et al. Chemical characterization and quantification of

proteoglycans in human post-burn hypertrophic and mature scars. Clin Sci (Lond) 1996;90(5): 417–25.

139. Zhang G, Ezura Y, Chervoneva I, et al. Decorin regulates assembly of collagen fibrils and acquisition of biomechanical properties during tendon development. J Cell Biochem 2006;98(6): 1436–49.

140. Raspanti M, Viola M, Sonaggere M, et al. Collagen fibril structure is affected by collagen concentration and decorin. Biomacromolecules 2007;8(7): 2087–91.

141. Zhang Z, Li X-J, Liu Y, et al. Recombinant human decorin inhibits cell proliferation and downregulates TGF-beta1 production in hypertrophic scar fibroblasts. Burns 2007;33(5):634–41.

142. Yamaguchi Y, Mann DM, Ruoslahti E. Negative regulation of transforming growth factor-beta by the proteoglycan decorin. Nature 1990;346(6281): 281–4.

143. Logan A, Baird A, Berry M. Decorin attenuates gliotic scar formation in the rat cerebral hemisphere. Exp Neurol 1999;159(2):504–10.

144. Kolb M, Margetts PJ, Galt T, et al. Transient transgene expression of decorin in the lung reduces the fibrotic response to bleomycin. Am J Respir Crit Care Med 2001;163(3 Pt 1):770–7.

145. Bittner K, Liszio C, Blumberg P, et al. Modulation of collagen gel contraction by decorin. Biochem J 1996;314(Pt 1):159–66.

146. Ferdous Z, Wei VM, Iozzo R, et al. Decorin-transforming growth factor-b interaction regulates matrix organization and mechanical characteristics of three-dimensional collagen matrices. J Biol Chem 2007;282(49):35887–98.

147. Tredget EE. Pathophysiology and treatment of fibroproliferative disorders following thermal injury. Ann N Y Acad Sci 1999;888:165–82.

148. Catty RH. Healing and contraction of experimental full-thickness wounds in the human. Br J Surg 1965;52:542–8.

149. Ramirez AT, Soroff HS, Schwartz MS, et al. Experimental wound healing in man. Surg Gynecol Obstet 1969;128(2):283–93.

150. Ramos ML, Gragnani A, Ferreira LM. Is there an ideal animal model to study hypertrophic scarring? J Burn Care Res 2008;29(2):363–8.

151. Carlson MA, Longaker MT. The fibroblast-populated collagen matrix as a model of wound healing: a review of the evidence. Wound Repair Regen 2004;12(2):134–47.

152. Ryan GB, Cliff WJ, Gabbiani G, et al. Myofibroblasts in human granulation tissue. Hum Pathol 1974;5(1):55–67.

153. Scott PG, Ghahary A, Chambers M, et al. Biological basis of hypertrophic scarring. Adv Struct Biol 1994;3:157–202.

154. Harris AK, Stopak D, Wild P. Fibroblast traction as a mechanism for collagen morphogenesis. Nature 1981;290(5803):249–51.

155. Harris AK, Wild P, Stopak D. Silicone rubber substrata: a new wrinkle in the study of cell locomotion. Science 1980;208(4440):177–9.

156. Ehrlich HP. Wound closure: evidence of cooperation between fibroblasts and collagen matrix. Eye 1988;2(Pt 2):149–57.

157. Squier CA. The effect of stretching on formation of myofibroblasts in mouse skin. Cell Tissue Res 1981;220(2):325–35.

158. Bell E, Ivarsson B, Merrill C. Production of a tissue-like structure by contraction of collagen lattices by human fibroblasts of different proliferative potential in vitro. Proc Natl Acad Sci U S A 1979;76(3):1274–8.

159. Nishiyama T, Tominaga N, Nakajima K, et al. Quantitative evaluation of the factors affecting the process of fibroblast-mediated collagen gel contraction by separating the process into three phases. Coll Relat Res 1988;8(3):259–73.

160. Tomasek JJ, Hay ED. Analysis of the role of microfilaments and microtubules in acquisition of bipolarity and elongation of fibroblasts in hydrated collagen gels. J Cell Biol 1984;99(2):536–49.

161. Buttle DJ, Ehrlich HP. Comparative studies of collagen lattice contraction utilizing a normal and a transformed cell line. J Cell Physiol 1983;116(2):159–66.

162. Delvoye P, Mauch C, Krieg T, et al. Contraction of collagen lattices by fibroblasts from patients and animals with heritable disorders of connective tissue. Br J Dermatol 1986;115(2):139–46.

163. Ehrlich HP, Rajaratnam JB. Cell locomotion forces versus cell contraction forces for collagen lattice contraction: an in vitro model of wound contraction. Tissue Cell 1990;22(4):407–17.

164. Montesano R, Orci L. Transforming growth factor beta stimulates collagen-matrix contraction by fibroblasts: implications for wound healing. Proc Natl Acad Sci U S A 1988;85(13):4894–7.

165. Reed MJ, Vernon RB, Abrass IB, et al. TGF-beta 1 induces the expression of type I collagen and SPARC, and enhances contraction of collagen gels, by fibroblasts from young and aged donors. J Cell Physiol 1994;158(1):169–79.

166. Clark RA, Folkvord JM, Hart CE, et al. Platelet isoforms of platelet-derived growth factor stimulate fibroblasts to contract collagen matrices. J Clin Invest 1989;84(3):1036–40.

167. Nedelec B, Shen YJ, Ghahary A, et al. The effect of interferon alpha 2b on the expression of cytoskeletal proteins in an in vitro model of wound contraction. J Lab Clin Med 1995;126(5):474–84.

168. Nedelec B, Dodd CM, Scott PG, et al. Effect of interferon-alpha2b on guinea pig wound closure and the expression of cytoskeletal proteins in vivo. Wound Repair Regen 1998;6(3):202–12.

169. Ehrlich HP. The modulation of contraction of fibroblast populated collagen lattices by types I, II, and III collagen. Tissue Cell 1988;20(1):47–50.

170. Ehrlich HP, Hembry RM. A comparative study of fibroblasts in healing freeze and burn injuries in rats. Am J Pathol 1984;117(2):218–24.

171. Stone PA, Madden JW. Effect of primary and delayed split skin grafting on wound contraction. Surg Forum 1974;25(0):41–4.

172. Rudolph R. Inhibition of myofibroblasts by skin grafts. Plast Reconstr Surg 1979;63(4):473–80.

173. Desmouliere A, Redard M, Darby I, et al. Apoptosis mediates the decrease in cellularity during the transition between granulation tissue and scar. Am J Pathol 1995;146(1):56–66.

174. Garbin S, Pittet B, Montandon D, et al. Covering by a flap induces apoptosis of granulation tissue myofibroblasts and vascular cells. Wound Repair Regen 1996;4(2):244–51.

175. Shin D, Minn KW. The effect of myofibroblast on contracture of hypertrophic scar. Plast Reconstr Surg 2004;113(2):633–40.

176. Garner WL, Rittenberg T, Ehrlich HP, et al. Hypertrophic scar fibroblasts accelerate collagen gel contraction. Wound Repair Regen 1995;3(2): 185–91.

177. Derderian CA, Bastidas N, Lerman OZ, et al. Mechanical strain alters gene expression in an in vitro model of hypertrophic scarring. Ann Plast Surg 2005;55(1):69–75.

178. Larrabee WF Jr, East CA, Jaffe HS, et al. Intralesional interferon gamma treatment for keloids and hypertrophic scars. Arch Otolaryngol Head Neck Surg 1990;116(10):1159–62.

179. Macintyre L, Baird M. Pressure garments for use in the treatment of hypertrophic scars—a review of the problems associated with their use. Burns 2006;32(1):10–5.

180. Mustoe TA, Cooter RD, Gold MH, et al. International clinical recommendations on scar management. Plast Reconstr Surg 2002;110(2): 560–71.

181. Anzarut A, Olson J, Singh P, et al. The effectiveness of pressure garment therapy for the prevention of abnormal scarring after burn injury: a meta-analysis. J Plast Reconstr Aesthet Surg 2009;62(1): 77–84.

182. Perkins K, Davey RB, Wallis KA. Silicone gel: a new treatment for burn scars and contractures. Burns Incl Therm Inj 1983;9(3):201–4.

183. Mutalik S. Treatment of keloids and hypertrophic scars. Indian J Dermatol Venereol Leprol 2005; 71(1):3–8.

184. Mahnoush M. Effects of silicone gel on burn scars. Burns 1990;35(1):70–4.

185. Kamolz LP, Kitzinger HB, Karle B, et al. The treatment of hand burns. Burns 2008;35(3):327–37.

186. Prasad JK, Bowden ML, Thomson PD. A review of the reconstructive surgery needs of 3167 survivors of burn injury. Burns 1991;17(4):302–5.

187. Ketchum LD, Smith J, Robinson DW, et al. The treatment of hypertrophic scar, keloid and scar contracture by triamcinolone acetonide. Plast Reconstr Surg 1966;38(3):209–18.

188. Al-Attar A, Mess S, Thomassen JM, et al. Keloid pathogenesis and treatment. Plast Reconstr Surg 2006;117(1):286–300.

189. Berman B, Viera MH, Amini S, et al. Prevention and management of hypertrophic scars and keloids after burns in children. J Craniofac Surg 2008; 19(4):989–1006.

190. Atiyeh BS. Nonsurgical management of hypertrophic scars: evidence-based therapies, standard practices, and emerging methods. Aesthetic Plast Surg 2007;31(5):468–92 [discussion: 493–4].

191. Lama PJ, Fechtner RD. Antifibrotics and wound healing in glaucoma surgery. Surv Ophthalmol 2003;48(3):314–46.

192. Apikian M, Goodman G. Intralesional 5-fluorouracil in the treatment of keloid scars. Australas J Dermatol 2004;45(2):140–3.

193. Nandakumar DN, Koner BC, Vinayagamoorthi R, et al. Activation of NF-kappaB in lymphocytes and increase in serum immunoglobulin in hyperthyroidism: possible role of oxidative stress. Immunobiology 2008;213(5):409–15.

194. Fitzpatrick RE. Treatment of inflamed hypertrophic scars using intralesional 5-FU. Dermatol Surg 1999;25(3):224–32.

195. Oh CK, Son HS, Kwon YW, et al. Intralesional fluorouracil injection in infantile digital fibromatosis. Arch Dermatol 2005;141(5):549–50.

196. Chen MA, Davidson TM. Scar management: prevention and treatment strategies. Curr Opin Otolaryngol Head Neck Surg 2005;13(4):242–7.

197. Berman B, Villa AM, Ramirez CC. Novel opportunities in the treatment and prevention of scarring. J Cutan Med Surg 2004;8(Suppl 3):32–6.

198. Tredget EE, Wang R, Shen Q, et al. Transforming growth factor-beta mRNA and protein in hypertrophic scar tissues and fibroblasts: antagonism by IFN-alpha and IFN-gamma in vitro and in vivo. J Interferon Cytokine Res 2000;20(2):143–51.

199. Yokozeki M, Baba Y, Shimokawa H, et al. Interferon-gamma inhibits the myofibroblastic phenotype of rat palatal fibroblasts induced by transforming growth factor-beta1 in vitro. FEBS Lett 1999;442(1):61–4.

200. Higashi K, Inagaki Y, Fujimori K, et al. Interferon-gamma interferes with transforming growth factor-beta signaling through direct interaction of YB-1 with Smad3. J Biol Chem 2003;278(44): 43470–9.

201. Davison SP, Mess S, Kauffman LC, et al. Ineffective treatment of keloids with interferon alpha-2b. Plast Reconstr Surg 2006;117(1):247–52.
202. O'Kane S, Ferguson MW. Transforming growth factor beta and wound healing. Int J Biochem Cell Biol 1997;29(1):63–78.
203. Roberts AB. Transforming growth factor-beta: activity and efficacy in animal models of wound healing. Wound Repair Regen 1995;3(4):408–18.
204. Shah M, Foreman DM, Ferguson MW. Neutralisation of TGF-beta 1 and TGF-beta 2 or exogenous addition of TGF-beta 3 to cutaneous rat wounds reduces scarring. J Cell Sci 1995;108(Pt 3): 985–1002.
205. Durani P, Occleston N, O'Kane S, et al. Avotermin: a novel antiscarring agent. Int J Low Extrem Wounds 2008;7(3):160–8.
206. Ferguson MW, Duncan J, Bond J, et al. Prophylactic administration of avotermin for improvement of skin scarring: three double-blind, placebo-controlled, phase I/II studies. Lancet 2009; 373(9671):1264–74.
207. Lee KK, Mehrany K, Swanson NA. Surgical revision. Dermatol Clin 2005;23(1):141–50, vii.
208. Alster TS. Improvement of erythematous and hypertrophic scars by the 585-nm flashlamp-pumped pulsed dye laser. Ann Plast Surg 1994; 32(2):186–90.
209. Alster TS, Williams CM. Treatment of keloid sternotomy scars with 585 nm flashlamp-pumped pulsed-dye laser. Lancet 1995;345(8959):1198–200.
210. Bouzari N, Davis SC, Nouri K. Laser treatment of keloids and hypertrophic scars. Int J Dermatol 2007;46(1):80–8.
211. Har-Shai Y, Amar M, Sabo E. Intralesional cryotherapy for enhancing the involution of hypertrophic scars and keloids. Plast Reconstr Surg 2003; 111(6):1841–52.
212. Atiyeh BS, Gunn SW, Hayek SN. State of the art in burn treatment. World J Surg 2005;29(2): 131–48.
213. Wu Y, Wang J, Scott PG, et al. Bone marrow-derived stem cells in wound healing: a review. Wound Repair Regen 2007;15(Suppl 1):S18–26.
214. O'Connor NE, Mulliken JB, Banks-Schlegel S. Grafting of burns with cultured epithelium prepared from autologous epidermal cells. Lancet 1981;1(8211):75–8.
215. Seo YK, Song KY, Kim YJ, et al. Wound healing effect of acellular artificial dermis containing extracellular matrix secreted by human skin fibroblasts. Artif Organs 2007;31(7):509–20.
216. Sahota PS, Burn JL, Brown NJ, et al. Approaches to improve angiogenesis in tissue-engineered skin. Wound Repair Regen 2004; 12(6):635–42.
217. Kataoka K, Medina RJ, Kageyama T, et al. Participation of adult mouse bone marrow cells in reconstitution of skin. Am J Pathol 2003;163(4):1227–31.
218. Nakagawa H, Akita S, Fukui M, et al. Human mesenchymal stem cells successfully improve skin-substitute wound healing. Br J Dermatol 2005;153(1):29–36.

Rehabilitation of the Burned Hand

Merilyn L. Moore, PT[a],*, William S. Dewey, PT, CHT, OCS[b],
Reginald L. Richard, MS, PT[b]

KEYWORDS

- Burn hand deformities • Burn scar contracture
- Burn rehabilitation • Splinting the burned hand
- Range of motion • Hand therapy • Hand function

Hands are the most frequent sites of burn injury,[1] and proper management is essential to assure that optimal functional recovery is achieved. Although each hand represents less than 3% of the total body surface area, burns to the hand are considered serious injuries and should be referred to a burn center.[2] The thin, highly mobile dorsal skin, the sensory-enriched palmar skin, and the delicately balanced musculotendinous systems are all at risk with a hand burn. Successful management of the burned hand does not result simply from closing the wound. The hand is ranked as one of the three most frequent sites of burn scar contracture deformity.[3–5] The resulting loss of function from burns that include or are specific to the hands can have a devastating effect on the numerous life roles of the patient at any age.

When possible, burned hands are best treated by the entire burn center team, including physical and occupational therapists, with knowledge of burn wound healing and the potential problems that can be anticipated. This article outlines the principles of burn rehabilitation generally accepted in current burn center practice and is based more on the experience of the authors than on controlled comparative studies.

PROBLEMS TO ANTICIPATE

A thorough understanding of the effect of thermal injury on the structures of the hand can minimize or even avoid many burn-related problems. Some of the more commonly encountered complications after thermal hand injury include postburn edema, scar contracture, joint deformities, sensory impairment, loss of skin stability, and restricted functional use of the hand. A brief overview is given in this article. Other complications of thermal injury to the upper extremity that ultimately affect hand function are also considered.

Postburn Edema

An increase in vascular permeability coupled with a shift of fluids to the extravascular space should be anticipated following thermal injury. In superficial partial-thickness burns, minimal fluid is leaked into the extravascular space, and edema is minor and transient. In deep partial-thickness and full-thickness burns, edema is more severe (**Fig. 1**) and prolonged.[6] As edema increases during the first 72 hours postburn, so may the pressure within the compartments of the hand. Consequently, excessive intracompartmental hand and forearm pressures will impair arteriovenous and lymphatic function.[7]

Hand Deformities

There are several common burn hand deformities that can result from injury itself or the sequelae of injury.

Claw hand deformity

Claw hand can occur in the early postinjury period as a result of edema, tendon injury, or scar contracture. An immediate consequence of

[a] Rehabilitation Therapies and Burn Plastics Clinic, University of Washington Burn Center, Harborview Medical Center, Box 359835, 325 Ninth Avenue, Seattle, WA 98104, USA
[b] Army Burn Center, Burn Rehabilitation, United States Army Institute of Surgical Research, (SDEWEY), 3400 Rawley E. Chambers Avenue, Fort Sam Houston, TX 78234-6315, USA
* Corresponding author.
E-mail address: mlmoore@u.washington.edu (M.L. Moore).

hand.theclinics.com

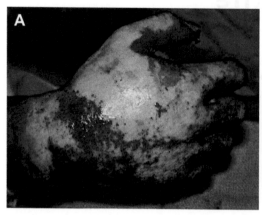
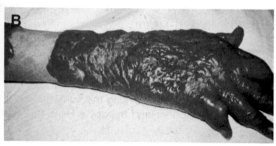

Fig. 1. Two complications of deep burn injury that can be minimized with intensive rehabilitation therapy include edema and scar. (*A*) Significant unresolved edema may result in limited mobility and chronic joint deformity. (*B*) Long-term hypertrophic scar that has not been molded and elongated to maximum length during its development is devastating, with permanent shortening of structures and joint deformity.

postburn edema can be hyperextension of the metacarpophalangeal (MP) joints and flexion of the interphalangeal (IP) joints, which is commonly referred to as a claw hand deformity (**Fig. 2**A). The severity of these deformities seems to be edema-dependent. Hyperextension of the MP joints occurs as the dorsal skin is drawn taut by the fluid shift into the extravascular tissues and as the palmar arches flatten. Flexion of the proximal interphalangeal (PIP) joints follows as a result of this edema-imposed tension on the common digital extensor tendon system and concurrent hyperextension of the MP joints.[8,9] The predisposition for MP joint hyperextension deformity to occur is intensified when the dorsal surface of the hand is also burned. Hyperextension

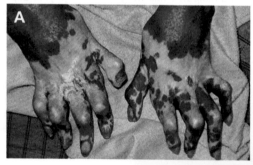
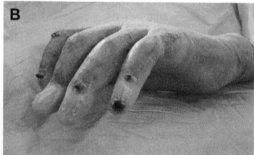

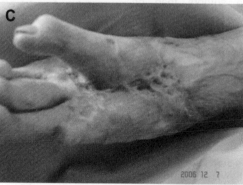

Fig. 2. Joint deformities can occur with tendon disruption, either from the original injury or from stretch or compression of damaged tendons. (*A*) Clawed hands with multiple deformities, including MP hyperextension, IP flexion, and thumb radial adduction. (*B*) Note boutonnière deformity of middle digit. (*C*) Palmar cupping deformity is frequently associated with hyperextension of the MP joint of the thumb, with loss of the grasping surface of the hand.

contractures of the MP joints may develop despite early surgical and well-planned therapy intervention, particularly in the presence of long-standing edema. The ring and little fingers account for 65% of problem digits, as studied by Graham and associates.[10]

Boutonnière deformity

The potential for this deformity is more likely with a deep burn involving the dorsum of the hand, fingers, or thumb. Boutonnière deformity in the fingers (see **Fig. 2**B) involves the extensor apparatus at the PIP joint level. This problem can be the result of direct thermal injury or of tendon ischemia. Tendon ischemia can result when the injured tendon is compressed between the eschar and the head of the proximal phalanx as the PIP joint is flexed.[11] The extent of damage to the extensor apparatus often is not known until inspected surgically.[12] In all deep partial-thickness and full-thickness burns involving the fingers and dorsal hand, because immediate surgery may not be feasible, involvement of the extensor apparatus should be assumed, and it should be protected until viability of the tendon system is known. An exposed tendon is at risk of desiccation and subsequent rupture, which will also result in a boutonnière deformity if it is located over the dorsal PIP joint. Therefore, it is recommended that all exposed tendons be kept moist and exposed tendons over the dorsal PIP joint be immobilized in extension until the tendon is no longer exposed. However, the distal interphalangeal (DIP) joint can be mobilized to allow lengthening of the oblique retinacular ligament (ORL). Later causes of a boutonnière deformity include flexion of the PIP joint secondary to scar banding in combination with a shortened ORL.[13]

Mallet and swan-neck deformities

Thermal injury to the terminal slip of the extensor tendon can result in loss of DIP joint extension or mallet deformity. Injury to the terminal slip can be a result of direct thermal injury or tendon ischemia induced as the injured tendon is compressed between the eschar and the base of the distal phalanx as the DIP joint is flexed.[14]

The swan-neck or PIP hyperextension deformity is characterized by hyperextension of the PIP joint and flexion of the DIP joint. The incidence of swan-neck deformity is most prominent in the middle finger.[15] Several causes for PIP joint hyperextension following burn injury have been hypothesized, including extensor digitorum communis tendon adherence, ischemic contracture of intrinsic muscles, joint stiffness from improper immobilization, and burn scar contracture.[15]

Palmar cupping deformity

The concavity of the hand's transverse and longitudinal palmar arches is accentuated in cupping-of-the-palm deformity (see **Fig. 2**C). Cupping of the palm can be anticipated when a burn is on the palmar surface of the hand, usually as a result of a contact burn. Precise evaluation of the depth of a palm burn in children is often difficult because the epidermis is very thin compared with the thickened calloused hand of an adult. Frequently the cupping deformity has a biomechanically associated hyperextension of the MP joint of the thumb. In addition to these deformities, sensory deficits and loss of the stable grasping surface of the palm should be anticipated. Palmar burns often require extensive therapy and multiple reconstructive efforts to yield functional results.[16]

Scar-band deformities

Scar bands develop when wounds cross lines of tension and run perpendicular to the axis of joint motion. These bands frequently cross multiple adjacent joints and are found at the borders of skin grafts and in areas that healed by secondary intention. Examples of common scar bands include the dorsal web spaces, the dorsal-lateral surfaces of the thumb and little finger, and the palmar surface of the fingers (**Fig. 3**). Loss of web space expansion creates considerable functional impairment. When the span of the first dorsal web space is shortened, thumb palmar abduction and circumduction are limited, and the thumb cannot be positioned away from the plane of the palm for grasp. When the span of the web spaces between the fingers is decreased, finger abduction can be severely restricted. If the width of the transverse volar arch is reduced, MP joint extension can be restricted. Functionally, placement of the hand around objects that require spherical grasp and any activities that require a flattened hand are impaired. Thumb radial abduction can be affected if scar bands are present on the thenar region of the palm.

Loss of skin sensation

Permanent sensory deficits following thermal injury should be anticipated, with limited potential for improvement, in all hand burns involving the dermis. Hermanson and colleagues[17] studied recovery of sensation in the grafted hand for 2 to 3 years postburn and found the final quality of sensation to be established at 1 month postgrafting. Sensory loss may also occur with neurologic damage to the upper extremity from multiple causes, such as electrical injury, tension or compression to peripheral nerves from edema, or improper positioning. These sensory deficits can

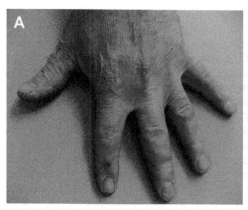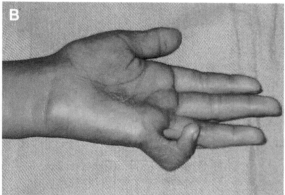

Fig. 3. (*A*) Scar bands of dorsal web spaces with resultant loss of web-space expansion may create functional impairment. (*B*) Palmar and lateral banding of the fifth digit results in flexion and ulnar deviation and places the distorted digit in the way of most hand activities.

affect overall hand function, including fine motor skills.

Fingernail deformities

Because dorsal hand burns are common, fingernails are involved and damaged frequently. Functionally, the fingernail acts as a rigid support against which the fleshy pulp of the finger can stabilize. This stability aids in sensation during pinch activities. Complete or partial loss of a fingernail is cosmetically disabling, and it may interfere with the stability of the fingertip. A burn that involves the surface of the fingertip often limits range of motion (ROM) of the DIP joint secondary to wound contraction.[18] These factors may contribute to problems with fine motor dexterity.

Peripheral nerve injuries

Peripheral nerve injuries tend to occur in association with high-voltage electrical injuries.[19–21] Neural tissue has a very low resistance to electric current and is particularly susceptible to injury. Hand function can be affected by both spinal cord injuries from current passing between contact sites around the spine and local nerve damage. Peripheral nerve damage is caused by direct influence of the current on the nerve and surrounding tissues and by swelling of an individual muscle compartment. Permanent damage to peripheral nerves, due to heat generated by current flow and immediate or delayed thrombosis of local vessels, is limited to the area of local tissue damage. The median and ulnar nerves are the most frequently injured nerves in electrical burns, reflecting the greater frequency of hand involvement in such injuries.[22,23]

Heterotopic ossification

Although heterotopic ossification (HO) is rarely seen in the hand, it is commonly seen at the elbow[24] in burn patients and can severely affect upper extremity function. This formation of new bone may occur in soft tissue surrounding the joint (**Fig. 4**) or within the joint capsule or ligaments, or it may form a bony bridge across the joint.[25] In some instances, this abnormal deposition of bone resolves spontaneously. In other cases, the continuous presence of HO limits the functional abilities of a patient so severely that surgical excision is necessary. HO is found more commonly in patients with a greater than 20% full-thickness burn and in patients whose wounds remain ungrafted for long periods of time.[26,27]

THERAPY MANAGEMENT GUIDELINES

Burn rehabilitation should be initiated within the first 24 hours of admission of a burn patient to establish an individualized positioning, splinting, exercise, and functional activity plan. Many of the complications previously described can be minimized with early and ongoing therapy. Patients with severe hand burns may require several years of scar management and reconstructive procedures that typically involve long-term rehabilitation. General guidelines for burn therapy approaches are outlined in the following sections.

Positioning

Specific positioning of the burned hand is crucial to healing with optimal results. Key components of positioning include elevating the distal extremity to facilitate venous blood flow, placing an elongation force on healing tissue, and protecting viable joint and soft tissue structures from additional trauma such as rupture or excessive pressure.

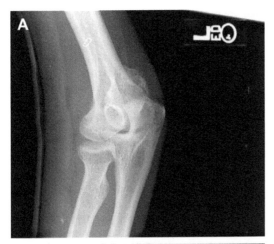

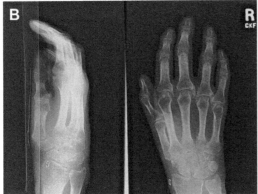

Fig. 4. HO is a common problematic complication in burn survivors. Although HO is not directly related to the hand burn injury, hand function can be greatly affected. (*A*) The elbow is the most frequent site of HO. (*B*) Although rare, bony deposits can occur at the small joints of the hand.

Edema management

Elevation of the hand and upper extremity is crucial to absorption of developing edema fluid. The hand should be elevated above heart level as much as possible. It is also critical to extend the elbow sufficiently to promote venous drainage. Various devices can be used to elevate the upper extremity, including pillows, foam wedges/ troughs, or slings, all supported on bedside attachments, intravenous poles, or furniture.

Secondly, a patient who is alert and able to participate should be instructed in active exercise to activate the muscle pump to decrease edema. The technique used to reduce edema should be selected carefully to avoid potential injury of fragile tissues. For example, frequent episodes of active composite finger flexion and extension can be encouraged safely in superficial partial-thickness hand burns. However, there is a risk of extensor tendon damage with passive composite flexion in

deeper hand burns. In these cases, exercises for isolated active or passive MP joint flexion, combined with active or passive IP joint extension, will impose less stress on this fragile extensor tendon system.[28] Repetitive finger abduction and adduction requires contraction of the dorsal and palmar interosseous muscles, which assists in edema reduction and is generally indicated for burns of all depths.[15] Edema control following the initial 72 hours should remain a priority to minimize stiffening of the soft tissue and loss of tendon glide and joint mobility.

Finally, edema control through externally applied pressure is frequently used in burn centers and thought to be clinically useful. Self-adherent elastic wraps have been proved to be effective on acutely burned and postoperative skin-grafted hands to control edema.[29] Hand edema measurements can be used to document improvement with elevation, motion, and compression. The figure-of-eight technique has proven to be a reliable and valid tool for measuring hand edema in patients with burns.[30] This technique is a more clinically feasible tool than water volumetry, which is considered the gold standard for hand edema assessment.[30]

Anticontracture positioning

As with any burned body part, the position of comfort for the patient becomes the position of contracture formation due to edema organization, wound bed contraction, and ultimate scar formation. The forearm frequently assumes a pronated position with the wrist in flexion when a patient elevates the forearm and hand or rests the segment on a pillow. If wrist ROM becomes limited in a specific direction, splinting the wrist in the opposite direction would be indicated. Circumferential forearm burns usually require the wrist to be positioned in slight extension due to the effects of gravity and the strength of the flexor muscles.

Positioning of the hand may vary from one therapist to another, but generally the antideformity position of the hand with a dorsal burn is an intrinsic plus position, consisting of wrist extension, MP joint flexion, PIP and DIP joint extension, and thumb palmar abduction.[31] This position combination can only be achieved by applying a custom-fit splint. If the IP joints are not deeply burned, wrapping a gauze roll or piece of foam into the palm and extending it through the thumb web space may provide adequate positioning. There is some controversy about whether the thumb should be positioned in radial or palmar abduction.[32] Whichever position is used, the objective is to preserve the thumb web space.

With deep palmar burns, the hand is usually positioned with all the finger joints extended and the volar thumb web space under stress to preserve finger extension and thumb radial abduction, respectively. These palmar burns need to be positioned by a splint. Following re-epithelialization, silicone elastomer may be added to the splint to provide positioning and scar management. With circumferential hand burns, the positioning program will need to be modified and alternated based on burn depth of each surface and the likelihood of scar contracture development.

Neuropathy prevention

The development of neuropathy is a common problem in patients with burns.[33] Specific areas that must be managed carefully to prevent nerve injury in the upper extremity are the shoulder for brachial plexus injuries, the elbow for ulnar nerve lesions, and the wrist for injuries to the ulnar or median nerves. A brachial plexus injury may result from improper positioning of the shoulder for prolonged periods of time. Shoulder abduction greater than 90° combined with external rotation decreases the distance between the clavicle and the first rib, which may result in compression of the plexus. This position, when combined with posterior displacement of the shoulder, may also cause stretching of the brachial plexus.[33] Placing the arm in scaption position, that is, midway between shoulder abduction and forward flexion and in neutral shoulder rotation, may relieve this compression.[34] Compression of the posterior cord of the brachial plexus by a splint or positioning device may result in a motor neuropathy in the radial nerve distribution.

Certain arm positions put the ulnar nerve at risk of compression as the nerve runs through the cubital tunnel at the elbow. When the elbow is flexed to 90°, the ulnar nerve is susceptible to pressure exerted by the arcuate ligament. When the forearm is pronated, the ulnar nerve is susceptible to an external compression force created by the surface on which the nerve lies.[33] The combination of these 2 positions puts the nerve doubly at risk. Ulnar neuropathy can be prevented by positioning the elbow in extension with the forearm supinated and positions alternated for comfort. Ulnar and median nerve involvement may be a result of compression at the wrist caused by extreme positions or excessive pressure.

Exercise and Activities of Daily Living

Skin biomechanics

Skin is a highly extensible tissue when compared with burn scar.[35] The skin overlying the dorsum of the hand and fingers is especially flexible with reservoirs of skin overlying the IP joints.[36] When making a fist, skin is recruited in a distal to proximal direction. Researchers have documented a 30% increase in finger length when moving from a position of total finger extension to complete fisting.[36] The joints of the fingers do not move like a door hinge; rather, the phalanx articulates around the head of the antecedent segment to account for the increase in finger length.

Range of motion

Emphasis is placed on the movements that oppose the development of contractures. The choice of exercise should be tailored to the individual needs of the patient. Active ROM is preferred to passive ROM (PROM); however, if patients are unable to achieve full ROM or participate with maximum effort, active-assisted movement or passive movement of the hand needs to be implemented. Alert patients can be taught self-range to ensure full combined tissue elongation (**Fig. 5**). PROM in the operating room, before excision and grafting procedures, enables the therapist to assess ROM restrictions and perform pain-free lengthening of tight structures.

The presence of multiple articulations within the hand makes it particularly susceptible to joint and scar contractures. To avoid joint contracture, it is recommended that ROM be performed to isolated joints before composite ROM. Composite ROM is required to provide maximal tissue elongation and prevent scar contracture of the hand.

Frequent exercise, performed multiple times throughout the day, is considered more beneficial than one intense session. Wound and scar contraction is a process that is ongoing throughout the day and night and this process needs to be treated constantly. Repeated ROM is helpful in mobilizing edema and preconditioning the tissue,[37,38] followed by sustained stress to elongate the scar as described later. Evaluations should be performed with the wound and scar tissue exposed, so appropriate exercise programs can be determined. When possible, ROM should also be performed in the absence of dressings so that the tissue can be observed during exercise, and treatment intensity can be adjusted appropriately. Strengthening and conditioning programs should be implemented, along with specific ROM exercises, as soon as the patient is able to participate actively.

Following tissue preconditioning, splints (static, static-progressive, or dynamic) or casts can be used to positively influence further gains in scar tissue length and subsequent ROM. Static devices demonstrate the biomechanical principle of tissue

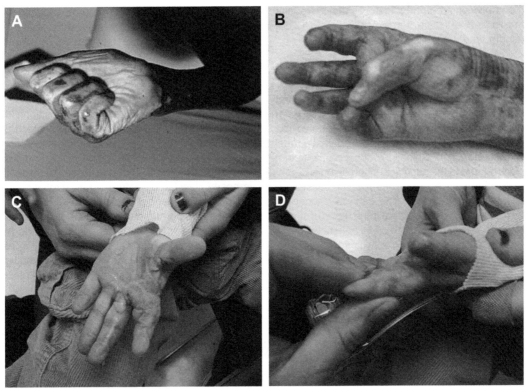

Fig. 5. ROM should be performed for maximum elongation of the healing skin or developing scar. (*A*) This can be achieved with active ROM in motivated alert patients. (*B*) Note blanching over thumb joints as opposition to the tip of the fifth digit is achieved, indicating maximum elongation of the scar. (*C*) It is difficult to obtain a full palmar expansion actively in the presence of developed scar. (*D*) Because this is a frequent injury in children, it is essential to instruct the child's parent/caregiver in appropriate techniques for passive ROM.

relaxation whereby tissue adapts to the stress applied. Dynamic interventions cause tissue to elongate over time.[38] By applying a constant load, tissue responds by increasing its length, which translates into increases in ROM.

Modalities

When the burn is closed and skin grafts are stable, modalities may be beneficial.

1. One recommended modality is paraffin, which provides moist heat and seems to soften skin/scar to promote increased ROM when used before exercise.[39] It is effective at lower temperatures, so it can be allowed to cool before applying to healed burn/scarred skin.
2. Scar massage may be helpful in reducing hypersensitivity, itch, and pain, and in moisturizing and softening of the scar for the duration of a treatment session, allowing easier and greater extensibility with ROM exercises and functional skills training.[40]

3. In addition to scar massage, other desensitization treatment is recommended when healed or scarred areas of the hand are hypersensitive, as evidenced by extreme discomfort or irritability in response to normally non-noxious tactile stimulation.[9] Desensitization techniques may include (1) dowel textures, with different textures of material glued onto dowel sticks; (2) contact, with use of particles such as rice and beans; and (3) vibration, with use of battery-operated vibrators.
4. The use of ultrasound has been reported in treating burn scar with limited success.[40]

Assistive devices

Age-appropriate self-care activities such as feeding, helping with dressing changes, bathing, applying moisturizing cream, and dressing are ways to increase physical activity.

Provision of simple aids such as built-up or extended handles and universal cuffs can facilitate independence; however, they should be implemented only if the patient has extraordinary edema or complicating comorbidities, as using regular utensils and self-care items can promote ROM, strength, and normalization of movement.

Splinting

Many splints have been described to treat hand burns based on the customized need of each patient.[41] Basic splinting principles should be directed toward elongation of tissue against normal wound contraction. Guidelines directing the use of splints related to the hand are based on burn depth, skin surface involved, burn rehabilitation phase, and patient considerations.[40] It is generally accepted that no splint is needed to treat hand burns of superficial partial-thickness depth or if a patient is able to maintain full active ROM. Prophylactic antideformity splinting of the hand at night may be helpful to prevent contracture following deep partial-

thickness and full-thickness burns. Splinting or other means of positioning after skin grafting to the hands is strongly recommended. A splint is also highly recommended for patients who are unable to actively maintain their own ROM, have a decreased level of consciousness, or are deemed uncooperative with treatment.[40]

The antideformity splint (**Fig. 6**) positions the wrist in extension, the MP joints in greater than 60° of flexion, and the IP joints in full extension.[42] This splint is recommended for any acute and post-acute burned hand that assumes the edema-imposed claw hand posture or has involvement of the common extensor tendons or extensor apparatus or has a burned area that includes the dorsum of the hand and digits. When skin coverage has been achieved, additional forms of splinting can be used to provide sustained stress across multiple joints. A composite flexion wrap (see **Fig. 6**) places

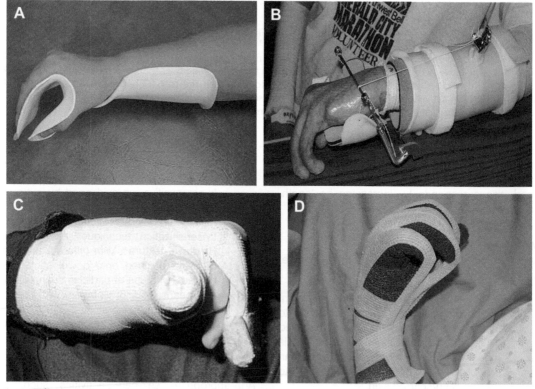

Fig. 6. Splinting can take many forms, indicated by individual patient need and stage of recovery. (*A*) A resting hand splint may provide adequate support for positioning the hand in the emergent and postgrafting period. If the extensor tendons are considered to be at risk, the IP joints are placed in full extension. (*B*) An example of dynamic wrist extension splint. (*C*) Casting may be required to fully hold joint position. This MCP block cast was aptly named the "shovel cast" by the 4-year-old patient, as he could still play in his sandbox while his new fifth finger dorsal graft healed. (*D*) Flexion wraps or straps can be useful in elongating dorsal skin/scar over IP joints or a combination of MP and IP joints. Strips of self-adherent wrap of a different color are applied over the wrapped hand, as tolerated for short intervals throughout the day.

maximum stress on the finger extensor mechanism, so it should be used only when the tendons are able to tolerate this force.

To successfully apply a sustained stress when the burn involves the palm and volar wrist, a splint should flatten the palmar arches and extend the digits. This position, however, places the MP joint collateral ligaments at their shortest length. In this situation, exercises to maintain collateral ligament length should be balanced with splinting to elongate the palmar wound or scar.

Pediatric considerations

In addition to the small size of children, the therapist must consider other anatomic differences, such as thinner, more fragile skin and hypermobile joints. Unlike adults and adolescents, small children do not tend to lose strength or joint mobility when immobilized in splints for extended periods, provided the splints are removed for regular exercise or activity sessions.

Some splints that work well with larger children or adolescents are not as effective with small children. For example, dynamic splints (see **Fig. 6**) are not recommended for small children because they are often difficult to keep in place. Serial static splints or casts (see **Fig. 6**) may be more practical and effective with smaller children. Because of a young child's small size, hand splints may have to be made longer so they can be anchored to an extended wrist; otherwise the splint will tend to slide distally and actually place the extremity in a deforming position. In addition, adding extra straps or applying the splint with an elastic bandage or self-adherent wrap may be necessary. Cotton socks over the splint may prevent the child from removing the splint.

Contact burns involving the palmar surface of the hand and fingers are common in toddlers.[43] The hand should be splinted in wrist extension and finger extension and abduction, with the thumb in radial abduction (**Fig. 7**). Splints should be worn all night and at nap time unless joint ROM is decreasing. Actions that can assist with desensitization and minimize palmar contractures include placing the palm and digits into extension,

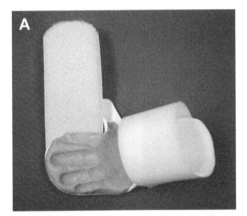
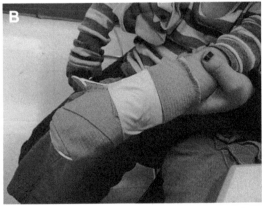
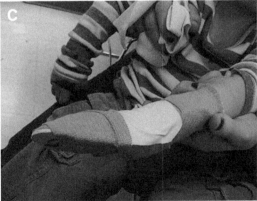

Fig. 7. Pan extension splint, useful in positioning palmar burns. (*A*) Elastomer putty insert can be custom molded and attached to the splint to apply pressure and full elongation within it. (*B*) and (*C*) Optimal positioning of this patient in the splint, with wrist and digit extension and thumb radial abduction. Note the need for overwrapping to keep the splint in place in a young child.

massage, and weight-bearing activities (eg, crawling on all fours or pushing a large heavy ball or toy).

Scar Management

Interim pressure

Early pressure application over the hand and digits can be accomplished by the use of thin, elastic self-adherent wraps (**Fig. 8**). This form of pressure aids in the early scar management of hands when the shearing force of donning a glove cannot be tolerated. Self-adherent elastic wraps may be applied over the burn dressings or directly onto digits. Before ordering custom-fit gloves, the use of prefabricated interim pressure gloves, which are made from softer materials, introduce the burn patient to circumferential pressure and allow any remaining edema to subside.

Custom garments and inserts

In the intermediate and long-term phases, pressure is applied to minimize scar hypertrophy. Because scar maturation is a dynamic process, the clinician must periodically review the need for pressure therapy, the type of pressure, and the physical condition of the gloves and inserts. Pressure gloves are available commercially as either custom-made (see **Fig. 8**) or pre-sized. Ready-made tubular support or pre-sized elasticized nylon fabric gloves can be used initially. Ready-made gloves are ideal for the burned hand that does not tolerate pressure well, for use in the final phase of scar control when less pressure is required to keep the scar flat, or for the sole purpose of holding pressure inserts, such as web spacers, in position.

Pressure applied to hypertrophic scars by a garment may not be adequate because garments often do not conform or apply equal pressure to all areas.[44] Areas that most often require a pressure insert are digital web spaces (see **Fig. 8**), the palm, and volar and dorsal wrist creases. Pressure in the palm of the hand cannot be achieved adequately with only a glove or self-adherent dressing. An insert can be fashioned out of silicone elastomer or elastomer putty (see **Fig. 7**). In addition to inserts, modifications to

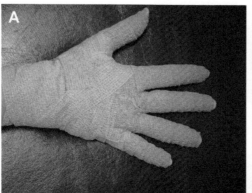
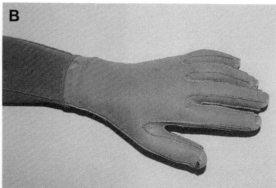
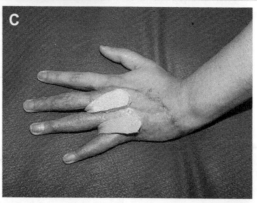

Fig. 8. Compression can facilitate edema reduction and scar alignment. (*A*) Self-adherent elastic wraps can be applied over dressings, providing early compression to reduce edema. (*B*) Custom-fit gloves provide long-term protection, support, and scar alignment. Note the slanted web-space design in this glove, included for specific compression of the dorsal web scars. (*C*) Further shaping and scar control is obtained with foam or inserts of other materials placed under the glove, in this case the third and fourth web-spaces.

pressure gloves can also facilitate wearing of the garment, particularly in enhancing function of the hand while wearing the glove.[45]

When compared with adults, young children appear to have a higher incidence of hypertrophic scarring and scar band formation, especially if the wound takes longer than 2 weeks to heal completely. Multiple garments should be ordered for children, and new garment measurements should be taken every 2 to 3 months or as needed to accommodate growth and development. Small hands are a challenge to measure and fit properly with pressure garments. For infants, better pressure on the hand may be achieved through the use of self-adherent elastic wraps. Narrow strips of foam padding, worn between the fingers under compression gloves, work well to preserve web spaces and do not macerate the skin or interfere with hand function. If a child's hand is burned only in the palm and does not involve the web spaces, a compression glove, used alone, is contraindicated—gloves tend to pull the thumb into adduction and fold the palm. Instead, a custom molded insert of silicone putty attached to a palmar extension splint is recommended.

Patient and Family Education

Therapy should be constantly directed toward patients' assumption of their own care. It makes no sense for the patient to receive one session of therapy followed by 23 hours of indifference and inactivity. Therefore home programs for which directives are clearly outlined are an essential part of treatment.[9] Educating the patient and family is very important in gaining the patient's trust, which promotes compliance and motivation. Written instructions with illustrations, frequent observation of therapy sessions combined with participation, and reciprocal demonstration of rehabilitation techniques, all help to ensure successful skill acquisition by a family member. Before discharge, the patient's rehabilitation program should be well established without daily changes. Patients or caregivers should be taught independence in handling wound care, proper application of splints, pressure garments and devices, and exercise and scar massage programs. A school-aged child should be prepared for return to school and association with friends, especially if functional loss or disfigurement has occurred. In addition to specific therapy techniques, two other topics are important for the team to share with patients and families: how to manage itch and sun exposure.

Loss or damage to sebaceous glands and sweat ducts tends to leave the skin dry and itchy. Instructing the patient in alternate techniques to scratching is important; examples include applying manual spot pressure or tapping the irritated area, applying a cold wet washcloth, frequently using a perfume-free and alcohol-free moisturizer, and using mild soaps and laundry detergents. Newly healed skin is prone to hyperpigmentation, so exposed areas such as the hands and arms should be protected from direct sunlight with clothing and routine use of a sunscreen (sun protection factor ≥30) even under pressure garments.

Outpatient Therapy

Frequently, patients with significant hand burns require ongoing hand therapy, following discharge from the burn center, to progress their ROM, strength, dexterity, and functional skills. The therapy needed may vary from 30- to 60-minute sessions 2 to 3 times a week to 4- to 8-hour work conditioning/hardening programs. In each case, communicating therapy outcomes and concerns with the referring burn center facilitates progression in therapy management and return to work/school/community activities.

Functional Outcome

Many hand evaluations are available, but no consensus has been reached on a battery of tests best suited to determine outcome of the burned hand.[46–48] The traditional methods of assessment are ROM and grip strength, but it is important to assess an individual's ability to actually use their hands. The shifting focus of health care outcomes acknowledges the importance of patients' perceptions of their medical treatments and the effects on their quality of life. In a recent study,[49] the Michigan Hand Outcomes Questionnaire revealed that 68% of patients reported hand function deterioration, 65% with the nondominant hand. Activities of daily living (76%) and work (59%) were the most affected.

In a large retrospective study of acute hand burns, Sheridan and colleagues[50] reported normal function in 97% of patients with superficial injuries and 81% of patients with deep dermal and full-thickness injuries requiring surgery. Although only 9% of those with injuries involving the extensor mechanism, joint capsule, or bone had normal functional outcomes, 90% were able to perform activities of daily living independently. In a review of deep (fourth-degree) hand burns from the 1980s, Nuchtern and colleagues[51] note that it took an average time of 13.3 months to return to work, with two-thirds of the patients changing their jobs in some way because of their hand impairment.

Long-term Follow-up

Most burn scars mature completely in 12 to 24 months, although skin changes can be observed for several years following a burn injury. It is possible to mold/influence scar tissue during this time, so it is helpful to provide the patient with intermittent visits to a burn specialty clinic to modify scar management techniques or plan timely surgical procedures for best outcome.

Long-term outpatient follow-up is necessary for a burned child to ensure maximum function and minimal cosmetic defect over the multiple growth periods between infancy and adulthood. Over a period of years, scars may interfere with normal growth, and a child may require additional surgery and therapy even after the scars are mature.

SUMMARY

Rehabilitation of the burned hand is challenging but vital in minimizing functional deficits. Burn rehabilitation therapists provide ongoing assessment and management of edema, burn scar contractures, and hand function. Therapy plans include positioning, splinting, exercise, compression, and functional skills training. These efforts are facilitated by experienced burn team members working together with common goals identified by the patient or caregiver. Therapy is most beneficial when started at the time of admission and may be needed for weeks or months following discharge. This article provides an overview of the role of burn rehabilitation therapy in the management of the burned hand.

REFERENCES

1. Smith MA, Munster AM, Spence RJ. Burns of the hand and upper limb: a review. Burns 1998;24:493–505.
2. Available at: http://ameriburn.org/BurnCenterReferralCriteria.pdf. Accessed July 22, 2009.
3. Dobbs ER, Curreri PW. Burns: analysis of results of physical therapy in 681 patients. J Trauma 1972;12:242–8.
4. Kraemer MD, Jones T, Deitch EA. Burn contractures: incidence, predisposing factors, and results of surgical therapy. J Burn Care Rehabil 1988;9:261–5.
5. Schneider JC, Holavanahalli R, Helm P, et al. Contractures in burn injury part II: investigating joints of the hand. J Burn Care Res 2008;29:606–13.
6. Witte CL, Witte MH, Dumont AE. Significance of protein in edema fluid. Lymphology 1971;4:29–31.
7. Salisbury RE, Dingeldein GP. The burned hand and upper extremity. In: Green DP, editor, Operative hand surgery, vol. 1. New York: Churchill Livingstone; 1982. p. 1523.
8. Littler J.G.W. The digital extensor-flexor mechanism. In: Converse JM, editor. Reconstructive plastic surgery, 2nd edition, vol. 6. Philadelphia: WB Saunders; 1977. p. 3166.
9. Hunter JW, Mackin EJ. Edema and bandaging. In: Hunter JW, Schneider LH, Mackin EJ, et al, editors. Rehabilitation of the hand. 3rd edition. St. Louis(MO): CV Mosby; 1990. p. 187.
10. Graham TJ, Stern PJ, True MS. Classification and treatment of postburn metacarpophalangeal extension contractures in children. J Hand Surg 1990;15A:450–6.
11. Maisels DO. The middle slip or boutonnière deformity in burned hands. Br J Plast Surg 1965;18:117–29.
12. Hunt JL, Sato RM. Early excision of full-thickness hand and digit burns: factors affecting morbidity. J Trauma 1982;22:414.
13. Valentin P. Physiology of extension of the fingers. In: Tubiana R, editor. The hand, vol. 1. Philadelphia: WB Saunders; 1981. p. 389.
14. Sherif MM, Boswick JA. Postburn proximal interphalangeal joint hyperextension deformity of the fingers. Bull Clin Rev Burn Inj 1985;3:32–5.
15. Wright Howell J. Management of the burned hand. In: Richard RL, Staley MJ, editors. Burn care and rehabilitation principles and practice. Philadelphia: FA Davis; 1994. p. 531–75.
16. Warden GD. The pediatric burn patient: issues in wound management. In: Boots burn management report, vol. 1. Lincolnshire(IL): Boots Pharmaceuticals; 1991.
17. Hermanson A, Jonsson CE, Lindblom U. Sensibility after burn injury. Clin Physiol 1986;6:507.
18. Donelan MB. Nailfold reconstruction for correction of postburn fingernail deformities [abstract]. Proc Am Burn Assoc 1991;23:142.
19. Henderson B, Koepke GH, Feller I. Peripheral polyneuropathy among patients with burns. Arch Phys Med Rehabil 1971;52:149–51.
20. Helm PA, Johnson ER, Carlton AM. Peripheral neurological problems in acute burn patients. Burns Therm Inj 1977;3:122–5.
21. Esses SI, Peters WJ. Electrical burns: pathophysiology and complications. Can J Surg 1981;24:11–4.
22. Dutcher K, Johnson C. Neuromuscular and musculoskeletal complications. In: Richard RL, Staley MJ, editors. Burn care and rehabilitation principles and practice. Philadelphia: FA Davis; 1994. p. 576–602.
23. Hammond JS, Ward CG. High-voltage electrical injuries: management and outcome of 60 cases. Southampt Med J 1988;81:1351–2.
24. Hunt JL, Arnoldo BD, Kowalske K, et al. Heterotopic ossification revisited: a 21-year surgical experience. J Burn Care Res 2006;27:535–40.
25. Hoffer MM, Brody G, Ferlic F. Excision of heterotopic ossification about elbows in patients with thermal injury. J Trauma 1978;18:667–70.

26. Jay MS. Bone and joint changes following burn injury. Clin Pediatr 1981;20:734–6.
27. Klein MB, Logsetty S, Costa B, et al. Extended time to wound closure is associated with increased risk of heterotopic ossification of the elbow. J Burn Care Res 2007;28:447–50.
28. Tanigawa MC, O'Donnell OK, Graham PL. The burned hand: a physical therapy protocol. Phys Ther 1974;54:953–8.
29. Lowell M, Pirc P, Ward RS, et al. Effect of 3M Coban Self-Adherent Wraps on edema and function of the burned hand: a case study. J Burn Care Rehabil 2003;24:253–8.
30. Dewey WS, Hedman TL, Chapman TT, et al. The reliability and concurrent validity of the figure-of-eight method of measuring hand edema in patients with burns. J Burn Care Res 2007;28:157–62.
31. Pullium GF. Splinting and positioning. In: Fisher SV, Helm PA, editors. Comprehensive rehabilitation of burns. Baltimore(MD): Williams and Wilkins; 1984. p. 64–95.
32. Apfel LM, Irwin CP, Staley MJ, et al. Approaches to positioning the burn patient. In: Richard RL, Staley MJ, editors. Burn care and rehabilitation principles and practice. Philadelphia: FA Davis; 1994. p. 221–41.
33. Helm PA. Neuromuscular considerations. In: Fisher SV, Helm PA, editors. Comprehensive rehabilitation of burns. Baltimore(MD): Williams and Wilkins; 1984. p. 235–41.
34. Jackson L, Keats AS. Mechanism of brachial plexus palsy following anesthesia. Anesthesiology 1965;26: 190–4.
35. Bartell TH, Monafo WW, Mustoe TA. A new instrument for serial measurements of elasticity in hypertrophic scar. J Burn Care Rehabil 1988;9:657–60.
36. Richard RL, Lester ME, Miller SF, et al. Identification of cutaneous functional units (CFUs) related to burn scar contracture development. J Burn Care Res 2009;30:625–31.
37. Richard RL, Miller SF, Finley RK Jr, et al. A comparison of the effect of passive exercise versus static wrapping on finger range of motion in the burned hand. J Burn Care Rehabil 1987;8:576–8.
38. Richard RL, Staley MJ. Biophysical aspects of normal skin and burn scar. In: Richard RL, Staley MJ, editors. Burn care and rehabilitation principles and practice. Philadelphia: FA Davis; 1994. p. 49–69.
39. Kowalske K, Holavanahalli R, Hynan L, et al. A randomized-controlled study of the effectiveness of paraffin and sustained stretch in treatment of burn contractures [abstract]. J Burn Care Rehabil 2003; 24:S67.
40. Richard R, Baryza MJ, Carr JA, et al. Burn rehabilitation and research: proceedings of a consensus summit. J Burn Care Res 2009;30:543–73.
41. Richard R, Chapman T, Dougherty M, et al. An atlas and compendium of burn splints. San Antonio (TX): Reg Richard, Inc; 2005.
42. Richard R, Staley M, Daugherty MB, et al. The wide variety of designs for dorsal hand burn splints. J Burn Care Rehabil 1994;15:275–80.
43. Scott JR, Costa BA, Gibran NS, et al. Pediatric palm contact burns: a ten-year review. J Burn Care Res 2008;29:614–8.
44. Mann R, Yeong EK, Moore M, et al. Do custom-fitted pressure garments provide adequate pressure. J Burn Care Rehabil 1997;18:247–9.
45. O'Brien KA, Weinstock-Zlotnick G, Hunter H, et al. Comparison of positive pressure gloves on hand function in adults with burns. J Burn Care Res 2006;27:339–44.
46. Esselman PC, Thombs BD, Magyar-Russell G, et al. Burn rehabilitation: state of the science. Am J Phys Med Rehabil 2006;85:383–413.
47. Chapman TT, Richard RL, Hedman TL, et al. Combat casualty hand burns: evaluating impairment and disability during recovery. J Hand Ther 2008;21: 150–8 [quiz 9].
48. Simons M, King S, Edgar D. Occupational therapy and physiotherapy for the patient with burns: principles and management guidelines. J Burn Care Rehabil 2003;24:323–35 [discussion: 2].
49. Umraw N, Chan Y, Gomez M, et al. Effective hand function assessment after burn injuries. J Burn Care Rehabil 2004;25:134–9.
50. Sheridan RL, Hurley J, Smith MA, et al. The acutely burned hand: management and outcome based on a ten-year experience with 1047 acute hand burns. J Trauma 1995;38(3):406–11.
51. Nuchtern JG, Engrav LH, Nakamura DY, et al. Treatment of fourth-degree hand burns. J Burn Care Rehabil 1995;16:36–42.

Reconstruction of the Pediatric Burned Hand

Robert L. McCauley, MD[a,b,*]

KEYWORDS

- Burned hands • Grafts • Flaps
- Osteocutaneous transfers • Distraction lengthening

The incidence of hand burn has been extensively reported.[1–5] Tredget[4] reported more than 1700 burns during a 10-year period. In patients with a mean total body surface area burn of 15%, 54% of the patients sustained burns to the hand and upper extremity. However, 75% of the burned hands were noted in patients with less than 20% total body surface area burns. Yet, the importance of the severity of hand burn with functional outcome was not addressed until Sheridan and colleagues[5] reviewed 1047 burned hands. In this classification scheme, patients with category I injuries required no surgical intervention in the management of superficial partial-thickness burns; 97% of these patients demonstrated complete functional return. Patients with category II injuries required skin grafts for closure; 81% of these patients were able to achieve nearly complete functional recovery. Patients with the most severe injuries involving tendons, joints, or bone were assigned to category III; only 9% of patients were noted to have returned to normal function (**Tables 1** and **2**). Thus, it is clear that the initial management of the acute burned hand along with the depth of injury can affect functional outcome.

ACUTE BURNED HANDS

All methods for the management of the acutely burned hand have the same goal in mind—functional rehabilitation. Usually this is accomplished by controlling edema, reducing inflammation, and facilitating early mobilization. Edema is controlled by elevation of the hand above the heart. The inflammatory response is minimized by early debridement and prompt wound closure. As

a rule, wounds that will not heal within 14 days of injury may require operative intervention. Wounds that appear to heal within 14 day of injury are allowed to do so without significant hypertrophic scarring or loss of function. Early mobilization of the joints in the burn hand, with or without surgical intervention, ensures restoration of function[6,7] (**Fig. 1**).

RECONSTRUCTION OF THE BURN HAND

Reconstruction of the burned hand can be challenging. Optimal results depend on the extent and depth of soft tissue damage, the immediate postburn care, operative intervention, and subsequent physical therapy. Unfortunately, most of these factors may be out of the control of the reconstructive surgeon.[8] Whitson and Allen[9] summarized the factors that contribute to deformities of the hand as persistent edema, wound infection, poor positioning, prolonged immobilization, and delayed or inadequate skin coverage. Although successful acute management of the burned hand has reduced the need for subsequent reconstruction, burn scar contractures along with subsequent compromised hand functions still occur.[10,11] The majority of these cases may be related to the severity of the initial injury. However, some cases may have been prevented by appropriate acute care (**Table 3**).

Peacock and colleagues[12] noted that the need for secondary reconstructive procedures is decreased by proper attention to positioning and ranging of joints during the acute phase of wound care. The success rates of such procedures increase in direct proportion to the degree of motion preserved before reconstruction. Parry[8]

[a] University of Texas Medical Branch, 301 University Blvd Galveston, Texas 77555-0724, USA
[b] Shriners Hospitals for Children, 815 Market Street, Suite 708, Galveston, Texas, USA
* Corresponding author. Shriners Hospitals for Children, 815 Market Street, Suite 708, Galveston, Texas 77550.
E-mail address: rmccaule@utmb.edu

Hand Clin 25 (2009) 543–550
doi:10.1016/j.hcl.2009.06.011
0749-0712/09/$ – see front matter © 2009 Published by Elsevier Inc.

Table 1
Burn injury categories

Injury Category	Definition
I	Second-degree burn that healed without surgery
II	Deep burn that required surgery but did not involve
III	Deep burn involving bone and requiring Kirschner-wire fixation

Modified from McCauley RL, Asuku ME. Upper extremity burn reconstruction. In: Mathes SE, editor. Plastic surgery. Philadelphia: WB Saunders; 2000. p. 1–41; with permission.

Table 2
Burn outcome categories

Outcome Category	Definition
A	Normal function
B	Abnormal function but able to perform activities of daily living
C	Hand cannot perform activities of daily living, such as feeding and toileting

Modified from McCauley RL, Asuku ME. Upper extremity burn reconstruction. In: Mathes SE, editor. Plastic surgery. Philadelphia: WB Saunders; 2000. p. 1–41; with permission.

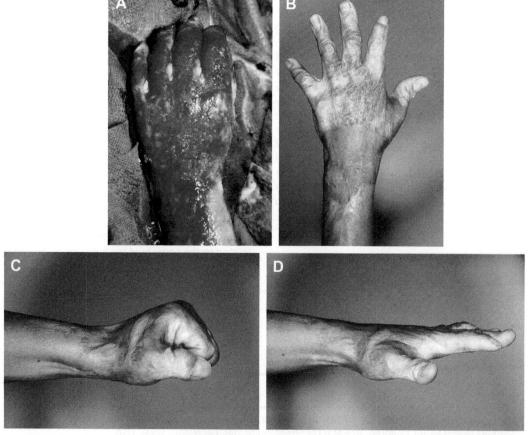

Fig. 1. (*A*) Early excision of a deep partial-thickness hand burn. (*B*) Result at 6 months after coverage with 1:1.5 unexpended meshed grafts. (*C*) Flexion at 6 months after coverage. (*D*) Extension at 6 months after coverage. (*From* McCauley RL, Asuku ME. Upper extremity burn reconstruction. In: Mathes SE, editor. Plastic surgery. Philadelphia: WB Saunders; 2000. p. 1–41; with permission.)

Table 3
Classification of burn scar contractures

Grade	Definition
I	Symptomatic tightness but no limitation in range of motion; normal architecture
II	Mild decrease in range of motion without significant impact on activities of daily living; no distortion of normal architecture
III	Functional deficit noted, with early changes in normal architecture of hand
A	Flexion contractures
B	Extension contractures
C	Combination of flexion and extension contractors
IV	Loss of hand function with significant distraction of normal architecture of the hand
A	Flexion contractures
B	Extension contractures
C	Combination of flexion and extension contractors

(*From* MCauley RL. Reconstruction of the pediatric burned hand. Hand Clin 2000;16(2):249–59; with permission)

noted that in the delayed evaluation of burned patients, reconstructive goals center on the restoration of function and form. Although many surgeons recognize the difficulties associated with the correction of burn-hand deformities, Donelan[13] observed that postburn hand deformities could be confusing to analyze because acute injuries and their methods of treatment vary so widely. In addition, multiple problems can exist in each postburn hand. However, Donelan was able to divide the deformities into three general categories. He noted that all of these categories might be present in a single hand: soft tissue deformities, joint deformities, and amputations.

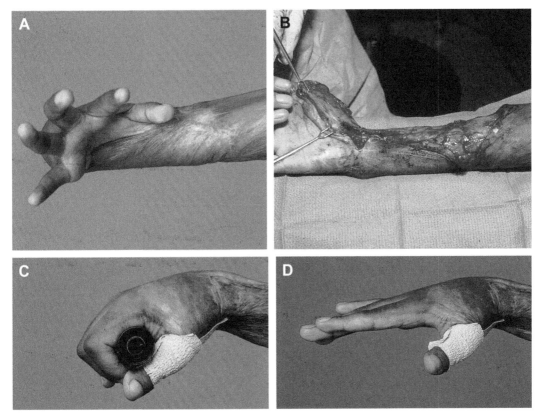

Fig. 2. (*A*) Severe radial volar contracture 2 years after burn injury. (*B*) Excisional release with subsequent coverage with a thick split-thickness skin graft. (*C* and *D*) Function 3 months after injury.

CLASSIFICATION AND MANAGEMENT OF BURN SCAR CONTRACTURES

Burn scar contractures are a major source of late morbidity in burn patients with burns over a large total body surface area. Restoration of function in patients with neglected contractures, while challenging, can be successful with skin flaps or free tissue transfer of skin flaps or fascial flaps.

The principles of reconstruction for correction of extreme dorsal contractures (grade IVB) are straightforward (**Figs. 2** and **3**):

1. Excise all scars such that anatomic restoration of the transverse and longitudinal arches of the hand is accomplished.
2. Kirschner wires for internal fixation with the metacarpophalangeal joints flexed to 80° to 90° and the interphalangeal joints at 180°.
3. Resurface the dorsum of the hand and fingers with skin grafts if the joints and tendons are protected; if joints are exposed, cover the exposed joints or tendons with flaps.

Severe volar contractures (grade IVA) may require excisional releases and resurfacing with

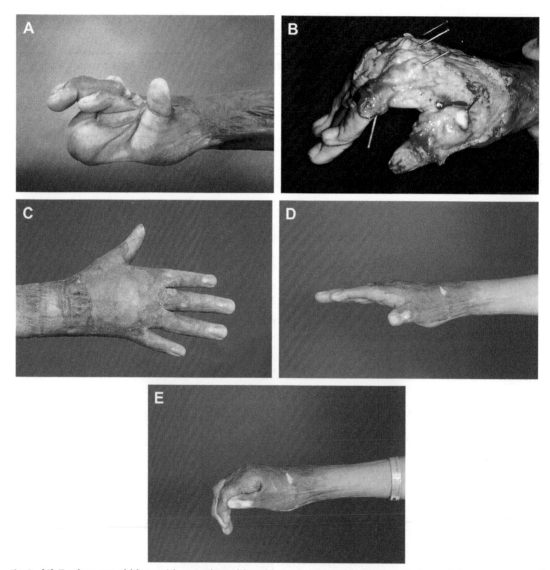

Fig. 3. (*A*) Twelve-year-old boy with a neglected hand burn 7 years after injury with loss of the transverse and longitudinal arches of the hand. (*B*) Excisional release with pinning of the metacarpophalangeal joints in flexion at 90°. (*C–E*) Appearance and function 2 months after coverage with a superficial temporal parietal fascial free flap and split-thickness skin graft. (*From* MCauley RL. Reconstruction of the pediatric burned hand. Hand Clin 2000;16(2):249–59; with permission.)

skin grafts or flaps. The metacarpophalangeal joints are kept in flexion to maximize the extent of the soft tissue release. In cases in which skin grafts are adequate for resurfacing the defect, cotton dressings in a tie-over bolster for immobilization are needed. Elevation of the affected part is important for successful graft take. Bolsters are removed on day five to seven postoperatively for inspection. Kirschner wires are usually left in place for 4 to 6 weeks. Unfortunately, many of these patients develop such contractures at a very young age and the time to reconstruction can be years after injury. Internal fixation of joints with Kirschner wires may be the only reliable source of splinting in very young patients. The functional outcome of these patients appears to be maximized with the use of Kirschner-wire fixation.

INTERDIGITAL CONTRACTURES

Burn syndactyly, or interdigital contractures, are a common sequela of hand burns involving the dorsum of the hand and digits.[14-16] Unless involving the first web space, interdigital contractures rarely cause significant functional deficits. Krizek and colleagues and others[15,16] reported that many of these problems may be corrected with a variety of local flaps, with or without the use of additional skin grafts. Functional problems can be significant if the first web space is involved. A number of techniques are available to maximize the use of local skin flaps (see **Fig. 3**). Mancoll and colleagues[16] reported the long-term follow-up of

various techniques used to surgically correct interdigital contractures. Although all techniques using skin grafts or local flaps showed a high recurrence rate, Z-plasties had the lowest recurrence rates.

DIGITAL LOSS

Patients who present with deep burns to the hand with digital involvement can be at risk for vascular compromise of the digits. Early escharotomy to preserve the intrinsic muscles of the hand and improve circulation of the digits is crucial. In spite of these maneuvers, however, some patients may face partial or total amputation of the digits. Such losses not only distort the appearance of the hand but can also hamper function. Reconstruction of the digits to improve function is frequently addressed with the thumb and index fingers. Littler[17] addressed the issue of thumb reconstruction in patients with multiple digital amputations by performing first-to-second metacarpal transfers using a vascularized osteocutaneous flaps. By combining two functionless digits to make a functional thumb, two improvements are achieved: (1) the thumb is lengthened and (2) a first-web space is developed, enabling pinching. Littler's patients were not burn victims. Even so, other surgeons have successfully applied this approach to the reconstruction of burned hands with digital amputations.[17-19] In patients with large total body surface area burns with involvement of the feet and multiple digital amputations, free toe-to-thumb transfers may not be possible. Thus,

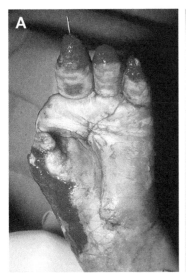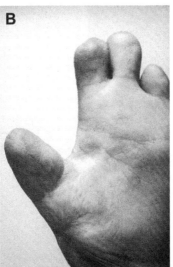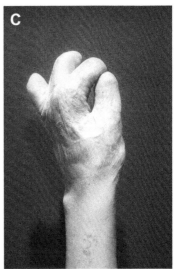

Fig. 4. (A) Five-year-old boy with full-thickness necrosis of digits, requiring partial amputation of the thumb, total amputation of the index finger at the proximal phalanx, and partial amputation of the third through the fifth digits. (B) Appearance after second-to-first metacarpal transfer to lengthen the thumb. (C) Key pinch demonstrated in the reconstructed hand. (*From* MCauley RL. Reconstruction of the pediatric burned hand. Hand Clin 2000;16(2):249–59; with permission.)

a careful analysis of the patient's overall condition allows proper consideration for metacarpal transfers in reconstruction of the thumb (**Fig. 4**).

An alternative to reconstruction of the burned hand with multiple digital losses involves the use of finger-lengthening techniques by distraction osteosynthesis.[20] As noted by Wainwright and Parks,[20] a corticotomy of the shortened digit is performed after placement of a mini-Hoffman

device for subsequent distraction. After 2 weeks, early callus formation occurs with immature woven bone and osteoprogenitor cells. Subsequent distraction of the healing callus can occur followed by a 2- to 4-week period of stabilization to allow the new bone to solidify (**Fig. 5**). The primary goal of this procedure is to restore pinch. Thus, the thumb and index fingers, if of adequate length, are the digits of primary interest.

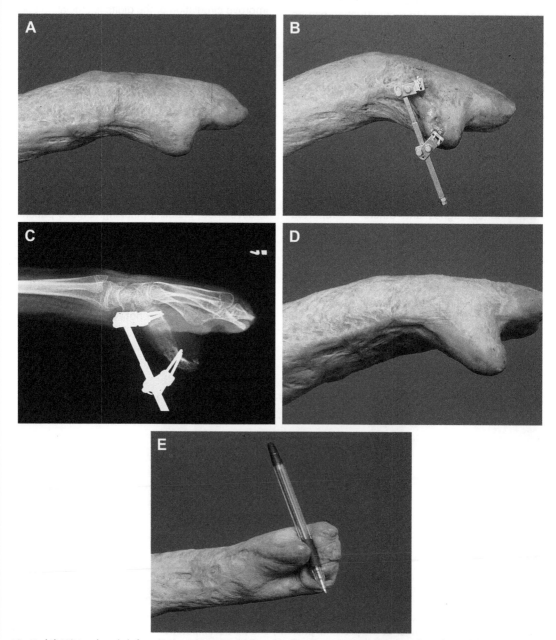

Fig. 5. (*A*) Mitten-hand deformity in a 10-year-old female after burn injury. The thumb is short. (*B*) Placement of a mini-Hoffman device for distraction lengthening of the thumb. (*C*) Radiograph shows 2.5-cm thumb lengthening. (*D* and *E*) Appearance and improved function after distraction lengthening of the thumb.

ELECTRICAL HAND BURNS

High-voltage (>1000 V) electrical injuries have an amputation rate of between 45% and 73%.[21] Total return of function in the upper extremities is low—approximately 6%—and no functional return has been documented in over 25% of patients. Consequently, presentation of the patients with viable but insensate hands after electrical injury is possible. Although, amputation is an option, reconstruction of the affected part should always be considered. Children who present with a viable, insensate extremity may require nerve reconstruction. Successful coaptation and regeneration of nerves require coverage with well-vascularized tissue above and below the nerve grafts. If the overlying tissue is scarred or otherwise inadequate, resurfacing of these areas with vascularized skin flaps is crucial. Once stable soft tissue coverage is obtained, reconstruction with sural nerve grafts can be accomplished. McCauley and colleagues[21] uniformly restored sensation in eight children with six extremities involved in electrical burns to the hands using sural nerve grafts to reconstruct the median and ulnar nerves up to 2 years after injury (**Fig. 6**). Needless to say, when nerve reconstruction is performed in a delayed fashion after extensive debridement of the forearm musculature, prognosis for the return of motor function is dismal.

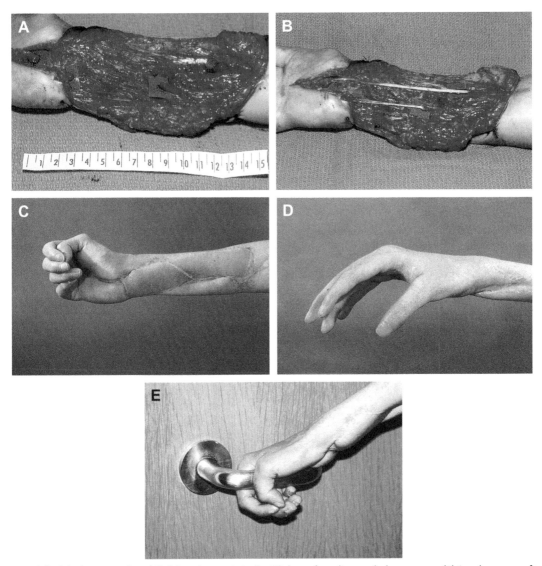

Fig. 6. (*A*) Right insensate hand (left hand amputated) with loss of median and ulnar nerves. (*B*) Sural nerve grafts used for reconstruction of median and ulnar nerves. (*C–E*) Subsequent function after reconstruction. (*From* MCauley RL. Reconstruction of the pediatric burned hand. Hand Clin 2000;16(2):249–59; with permission.)

Secondary procedures, such as tendon transfers and digital arthrodesis, may improve function once sensation has been reestablished.

SUMMARY

Reconstruction of pediatric hand burns can be a difficult task. Attention to details during the acute phase of injury may be the surgeon's greatest ally in functional rehabilitation of the burned hand. Reducing edema and inflammation, while maintaining digital circulation, and fostering early mobilization of the limb are keys to ensuring return of function. Patients burned in childhood may present with neglected contractures long after the burn took place. Surgical intervention can improve hand function. Loss of the thumb in children with large total body surface area burns can be approached reliably by lengthening of the thumb using first-to-second metacarpal transfers or distraction lengthening.[17,18,20] Although electrical injuries represent only a small fraction of patients admitted to hospitals, children who present with viable insensate hands may have sensory return more than 1 year after injury. Thus a more aggressive surgical approach to restore form and function may be required.

REFERENCES

1. American Burn Association. Guidelines for service standards and severity classification in the treatment of burn injury. Bull Am Coll Surg 1984;69:24–9.
2. American Medical Association. Guides to the evaluation of permanent impairment. 4th edition. Chicago (IL): American Medical Association; 1994.
3. Engrav LH, Dutcher KA, Nakamura KY. Rating burn impairment. Clin Plast Surg 1992;19:569–98.
4. Tredget E. Management of the acutely burned upper extremity. Hand Clin 2000;16:187–202.
5. Sheridan RL, Hurley J, Smith MA, et al. The acutely burned hand: management and outcome based on a ten-year experience with 1047 acute hand burns. J Trauma 1995;38:406–11.
6. Krizek TJ, Flagg SV, Wolfort FG, et al. Delayed primary excision and skin grafting of the burn hand. Plast Reconstr Surg 1973;51:524.
7. Robson MC, Smith DJ, Vandemer AJ, et al. Making the burn hand function. Clin Plast Surg 1992;19: 633–71.
8. Parry SW. Reconstruction of the burned hand. Clin Plast Surg 1989;16:577–86.
9. Whitson TC, Allen BD. Management of the burned hand. J Trauma 1971;11:606–9.
10. McCauley RL. Reconstruction of the pediatric burned hand. Hand Clin 2000;16:249–59.
11. Burns BF, McCauley RL, Murphy FL, et al. Reconstruction management of patients with greater than 80% TBSA burns. Burns 1993;19:429–33.
12. Peacock EE, Madden JW, Trier WC. Some studies on the treatment of the burned hand. Ann Surg 1970;171:903–8.
13. Donalon MB. Reconstruction of the burned hand and upper extremity. In: May JW Jr, Littler JW, editors. The hand. Philadelphia: W.B. Sanders; 1990. p. 5452–82.
14. Adamson JE, Crawford HH, Horton CE, et al. Treatment of dorsal burn adduction contractures of the hand. Plast Reconstr Surg 1968;42:355–9.
15. Krizek TJ, Robson MC, Flagg SV. Management of burn syndactyly. J Trauma 1974;14:587–93.
16. Mancoll JS, Mlakar JM, McCauley RL, et al. Burn web space contractures—are they just a bad penny? Proc Am Burn Assoc 1996;28:111.
17. Littler JW. The neurovascular pedicle method of digital transposition for reconstruction of the thumb. Plast Reconstr Surg 1953;12:303–19.
18. May JW, Donalon MB, Toth MD, et al. Thumb reconstruction in the burned hand by advancement pollicizations of the second ray remnant. J Hand Surg 1984;9:484–9.
19. Ward JW, Pensler JM, Parry SW. Pollicization of the thumb for reconstruction in severe pediatric hand burns. Plast Reconstr Surg 1985;76: 927–32.
20. Wainwright D, Parks DH. Finger lengthening of the burned hand by distraction osteosynthesis. In: McCauley RL, editor. Functional and aesthetic reconstruction of burned patients. New York: Taylor and Francis; 2005. p. 463–74.
21. Roberts L, Meyers R, Pierre E, et al. Sensory analysis of nerve grafting in children with electrical burns of the upper extremity. Proc Am Burn Assoc 1996; 27:123.

Microsurgical Reconstruction of the Burned Hand

Yvonne L. Karanas, MD[a,b,c],*, Rudolf F. Buntic, MD[c,d]

KEYWORDS

- Microsurgery • Hand burns
- Delayed hand burn reconstruction • Electrical injury
- Hand contracture

The severely burned hand is a catastrophic injury because of the potential loss of hand function and resulting disability. Elevation, splinting, dressing changes, and excision remain the principles of early management, with escharotomies and fasciotomies being performed as needed. Most hand burns can be treated successfully with skin grafts. However, despite appropriate initial management, some patients develop digital necrosis or have exposed bone, tendons, and nerves, requiring more than skin graft coverage. The use of free flaps allows the surgeon to bring in vascularized tissue to provide coverage of vital structures without the risk of contracture over time. As in acute reconstruction, most secondary reconstructions can be performed with local flaps or skin grafts. However, severe contractures, large unstable areas, and total digit reconstruction all require microsurgical correction to achieve optimal results. As experience with microsurgery in burn patients has increased, these procedures can be safely performed with good outcomes.

A wide variety of muscle, musculocutaneous, fasciocutaneous, and fascial flaps that can be used in acute and delayed burn reconstruction are now well described. Flap selection is based on desired tissue characteristics, donor site availability, length of flap pedicle, availability of recipient vessels, and patient and surgeon preference. Microvascular anastomosis should be performed outside the zone of injury to maximize success rates. This becomes particularly important in electrical injuries in which the zone of injury may be extensive. Donor site selection may be challenging in the burn patient, as often many areas have sustained thermal injuries and are not options for tissue transfer. The surgeon should also consider the need for additional skin grafts on the flap or donor site, because skin may be limited after major burns.

ACUTE THERMAL INJURIES

After initial management and resuscitation, early excision is performed for all third and fourth degree hand burns. Clearly nonviable tissue is removed. Questionable tissue may be left initially, then reevaluated and excised at a second-look procedure as needed. Once wound evolution is complete, the nature of the wound is examined. If tendons, bone, or nerves are exposed, skin graft coverage alone will be inadequate. Local, distant, and free flaps should be considered at this time. Given the differences in anatomy and function, there are different considerations in the management of dorsal and palmar injuries.

Dorsum of the Hand

The skin on the dorsum of the hand is thin and pliable, providing supple coverage of the underlying extensor tendons and bones. Coverage of

a Santa Clara Valley Medical Center, 751 South Bascom Avenue, San Jose, CA 95128, USA
b Burn Center, Santa Clara Valley Medical Center, 751 South Bascom Avenue, San Jose, CA 95128, USA
c Department of Surgery, Stanford University School of Medicine, 300 Pasteur Drive, Stanford, CA 94305, USA
d The Buncke Clinic, Davies Medical Center, 45 Castro Street, Suite 121, San Francisco, CA 94114, USA
* Corresponding author. Santa Clara Valley Medical Center, 751 South Bascom Avenue, San Jose, CA 95128.
E-mail address: ykaranas@gmail.com (Y.L. Karanas).

Hand Clin 25 (2009) 551–556
doi:10.1016/j.hcl.2009.06.009
0749-0712/09/$ – see front matter © 2009 Published by Elsevier Inc.

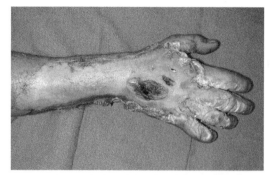

Fig. 1. Patient with dorsal hand and forearm burn.

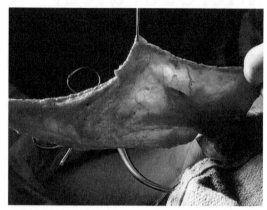

Fig. 4. The appearance of the thoracic fascia flap following elevation.

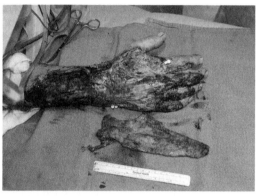

Fig. 2. Following excision, there were exposed extensor tendons.

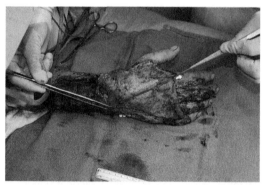

Fig. 5. Inset of flap showing coverage of exposed tendons with a thin fascial flap.

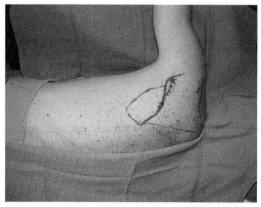

Fig. 3. Preoperative markings for a dorsal thoracic fascial flap.

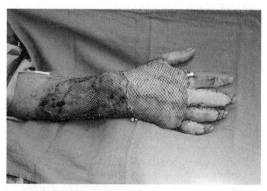

Fig. 6. Following inset of the flap, coverage is completed with a split thickness skin graft.

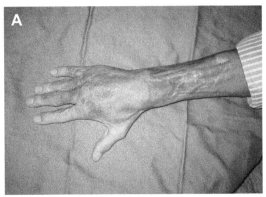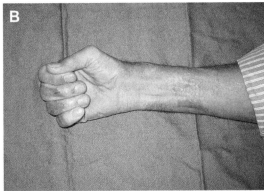

Fig. 7. (A) Postoperative result demonstrating a healed wound and (B) range of motion.

this area requires similar tissue. In the severely burned upper extremity, local flaps, consisting of reverse radial forearm flaps or posterior interosseous artery flaps, are often involved in the zone of injury and are therefore not available. Following the principle of "replacing like with like," we routinely use fascial or fasciocutaneous flaps for this area. Flap options include the contralateral radial forearm flap, anterolateral thigh flap, lateral arm flap, serratus fascia, dorsal thoracic fascia, dorsalis pedis flap, and temporoparietal fascial flap. All of these flaps provide thin pliable tissue to resurface the dorsum of the hand and allow for delayed tendon or bone reconstruction as needed. Most may be used as either fascial or fasciocutaneous flaps. The choice should be based on body habitus, size of the wound, necessary pedicle length to reach outside the zone of injury, and additional burns. In an obese patient, the standard anterolateral thigh flap may be thick. Consideration can be given to thinning the flap before inset.[1] The dorsalis pedis flap has been associated with donor site morbidity and may not be a good choice for patients with vascular disease of the lower extremity (**Figs. 1–7**).

Palmar Surface of the Hand

The palm represents a greater challenge because of the high functional demands placed on its skin. The palm has glabrous skin, which is thick, hairless, and anchored through complex fibrous septa. Fortunately, most palm burns will heal with conservative treatment, and only a small percentage require autografting.[2] Exposure of vital structures in the palm is rare after thermal injury and usually occurs in conjunction with extensive, severe burns or additional trauma. Thin fasciocutaneous flap, if available, will provide pliable tissue that can be reinnervated to enable sensory recovery (**Figs. 8–13**). The flap skin is not anchored

like the normal palmar skin and patients may have difficulty opening jars or doors as the skin may shift. Larger flaps may place too much bulk into the palm and limit the patient's ability to hold or grasp objects. Free flaps may also be used to resurface the palm if the patient has failed the more conservative treatment of skin grafting. The constant trauma that the palm sustains may cause skin graft breakdown, further inflammation, and scar contracture. In these cases, if local flaps are unavailable, microvascular reconstruction should be considered.

ELECTRICAL INJURIES

High-voltage electrical injuries commonly require microvascular reconstruction. These injuries frequently involve the hand and forearm as points of entry or contact. As with all high-voltage electrical injuries, the outer wound may only reveal a small fraction of the total destruction. Because of severe tissue destruction, limb salvage may be

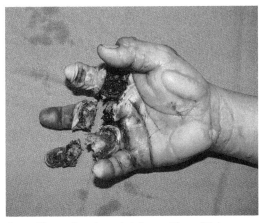

Fig. 8. Thermal and crush injury with multiple amputated digits.

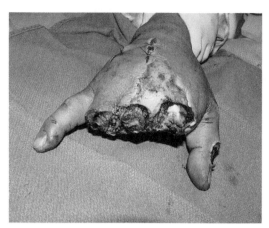

Fig. 9. After wound debridement, the metacarpals were exposed.

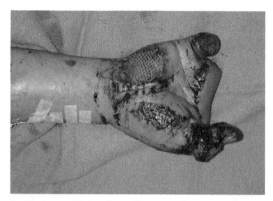

Fig. 11. Inset of lateral arm flap over the exposed metacarpal bones.

the primary goal in many of these patients. The muscles adjacent to the bones are commonly injured, as are nerves and blood vessels. Serial debridement is performed as needed until wound evolution is complete and all necrotic tissue has been excised. Various negative pressure wound therapy devices can be used as a temporary dressing to avoid desiccation of nerves, tendons, and bones until permanent coverage can be achieved. Large volumes of vascularized tissue are often needed to provide coverage and to fill any dead space that may be present around tendons or bones of the hand or forearm. Because of the large volume of tissue required and the need to fill dead space, free muscle flaps are routinely used in these patients (**Figs. 14–16**). Flap choice depends on the volume of tissue required, the need to fill dead space, the available donor sites, and the length of the vascular pedicle required. As vascular thrombosis is common with electrical injuries, vascular imaging is routinely obtained preoperatively for precise surgical planning. Research by Baumeister and colleagues[3] and

Sauerbier and colleagues[4] demonstrates that flap failure is higher in the acute reconstruction patient as compared with those undergoing delayed reconstruction. Free flaps performed between days 5 and 21 had the highest incidence of flap loss. Most free flaps performed in this period were for limb salvage, and surgery was therefore necessary at this time.

DELAYED RECONSTRUCTION
Unstable Wounds

Patients sustaining large TBSA (total body surface area) burns often have portions heal by secondary intention, or they have thinner, widely meshed grafts placed on their hands as skin may not be available for coverage. As the patients resume their activities, problems with wound breakdown in their hands may occur. Frequently, these will respond to local wound care. However, in a subset of patients the breakdown is chronic, leading to increasing inflammation and scar contracture. If

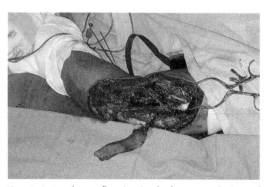

Fig. 10. Lateral arm flap in situ before completion of harvest.

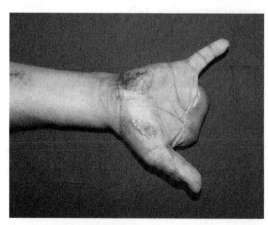

Fig. 12. Postoperative results demonstrating a healed wound.

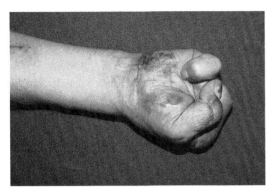

Fig. 13. Postoperative result demonstrating maximization of remaining hand function.

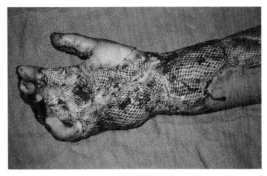

Fig. 15. Coverage of the forearm with a rectus flap and skin graft.

free tissue transfer is an option, the involved area is excised until healthy graft or normal tissue is reached, and all scar tissue has been removed. The entire area is then resurfaced with a free flap. If patients have unstable coverage and need additional reconstructive procedures on the underlying tendons, joints, or bones, the authors feel that free flap reconstruction is indicated, to provide primary wound healing and to allow for early range of motion if necessary. In these cases, the preference is for fasciocutaneous flaps where the donor site can be closed primarily so that no additional skin grafting is needed.

Hand Contractures

Despite appropriate initial management, graft and wound contracture can lead to significant hand contractures. Initial treatment consists of contracture release with local flaps or skin grafts as appropriate. Severe contractures or failures of more conservative procedures are candidates for free

flap reconstruction in conjunction with contracture release. Often, capsulotomies, volar plate release, tendon grafting, or check rein ligament releases are needed to release fixed joints. Stable coverage is needed over the joint to allow for movement after surgery. Free flaps may be necessary when joint or tendon exposure is anticipated after release or when the overlying scar is too unstable to tolerate surgical manipulations. Woo and Seul[5] reported 100% flap survival and improved functional outcomes in 18 patients with severe burn contractures after contracture release and free fasciocutaneous flap reconstruction. Uyger and colleagues[6] used the free medial pedis perforator flap to cover the palm and volar digits after flexion contracture release. Their data show an increase in MP joint extension postoperatively, with sensory reinnervation when neurorrhaphy was performed.

Substantial tissue loss or graft contracture can also result in a first web space contracture. Initial treatment includes contracture release, Z-plasties, and full-thickness grafts. If these are unsuccessful, free tissue transfer should be considered. Fasciocutaneous flaps can be used to resurface the web space and enable better opening of the hand. If

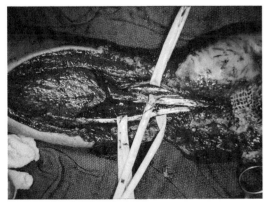

Fig. 14. This 19-year-old man sustained a high-voltage injury to his upper extremity. After debridement of all nonviable tissues, the tendons of the forearm are exposed.

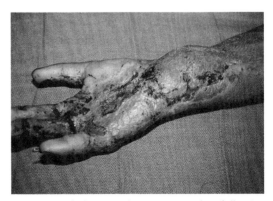

Fig. 16. Healed wounds at 4 weeks following reconstruction.

fasciocutaneous flaps are unavailable because of the prior burn, muscle flaps can be used and thinned at a secondary procedure.[7]

Toe Transfers

Severe hand burns may result in loss of one or even all digits. After initial treatment and hand therapy, hand function should be assessed. Patients with thumb loss or multiple digit loss may be candidates for toe transfers if their feet are not injured. These free tissue transfers can be reliably performed and can significantly improve the patients' overall hand function. Williamson and colleagues[8] showed substantial gains in hand function after toe to finger transfer in the fingerless patient. In extreme cases, with the loss of multiple digits and palmar or dorsal defects, wound coverage can be achieved with a fasciocutaneous or muscle flap. Once the patient's wounds have healed, toe transfers can be performed as a secondary procedure to improve hand function.

SUMMARY

Most routine hand burns can be managed without microsurgical techniques. Severe third and fourth degree hand burns or electrical injuries with exposure of nerves, tendons, or bones require microsurgical treatment if local tissue is insufficient or injured. Microsurgical reconstruction plays an important role in delayed reconstruction because it allows the surgeon to bring in vascularized tissue to scarred, unstable areas. Uncomplicated wound healing can occur over joint or tendon reconstruction and allow for early range of motion and healing with minimal contracture.

ACKNOWLEDGMENTS

We gratefully acknowledge Dr. Kenneth Yim for his assistance in digitizing photographs of Figures 14–16.

REFERENCES

1. Adani R, Tarallo L, Marcoccio I, et al. Hand reconstruction using the thin anterolateral thigh flap. Plast Reconstr Surg 2005;116:467–73.
2. Pensler JM, Steward R, Lewis SR, et al. Reconstruction of the burned palm: full-thickness versus split-thickness skin grafts–long-term follow-up. Plast Reconstr Surg 1988;81:46–9.
3. Baumeister S, Koller M, Dragu A, et al. Principles of microvascular reconstruction in burn and electrical burn injuries. Burns 2005;31:92–8.
4. Sauerbier M, Ofer N, Germann G, et al. Microvascular reconstruction in burn and electrical burn injuries of the severely traumatized upper extremity. Plast Reconstr Surg 2007;119:605.
5. Woo SH, Seul JH. Optimizing the correction of severe postburn hand deformities by using aggressive contracture releases and fasciocutaneous free-tissue transfers. Plast Reconstr Surg 2001;107:1–8.
6. Uygur F, Duman H, Ülkür E, et al. Chronic postburn palmar contractures reconstruction using the medial pedis perforator flap. Ann Plast Surg 2008;61(3):269–73.
7. Kalliainen LK, Schubert W. The management of web space contractures. Clin Plast Surg 2005;32:503–14.
8. Williamson JS, Manktelow RT, Kelly L, et al. Toe-to-finger transfer for post-traumatic reconstruction of the fingerless hand. Can J Surg 2001;44(4):275–83.

Outcome Assessment After Hand Burns

Karen Kowalske, MD

KEYWORDS

- Burns • Outcomes • Functional assessment
- Contractures • Employment

A review of the literature on outcome after hand burns produces a general impression that the outcome after partial and full hand burns is good to excellent and that outcome after deep full-thickness hand burns is universally poor. Clinical experience and a detailed review of the literature reinforces that this is not the whole picture. Determining and describing outcome after hand burn has not been well studied, but is clearly a difficult task because impairment measurements and functional hand tasks do not necessarily describe the individual patient experience. Also, assessing range of motion of the hand produces an overwhelming volume of data that is difficult to interpret. Is 30° loss of extension in the third digit equivalent to 30° loss of flexion in the fourth? Regarding this challenge, the literature on hand outcomes is less than satisfactory.

Long-term outcome after hand burn is typically influenced by several factors, including depth of burn, edema during the acute period, formation of hypertrophic scar, joint contracture, lack of compliance with therapy regimen, pain, and neuropathy. There have been few studies that provide a longitudinal assessment of hand function after burn injury, and most of the literature on long-term outcome after hand burns focuses on techniques for correction of scar contractures and not true functional outcome. In addition, few studies examine the best methods for assessing hand function. This article reviews descriptive studies, assessments of hand strength and range of motion, and community integration, in an effort to provide the reader with a better understanding of the current literature regarding hand burn outcome as well as the areas that are important for future investigation.

DESCRIPTIVE STUDIES

Most of the literature on hand burn outcome primarily comprises descriptive studies. There are enumerable studies of a single case or two cases with a description of a reconstructive surgical approach, which is not particularly useful in the discussion of population outcomes, so these studies are not be discussed in this article. There are a few large-scale studies looking at outcome after hand burn that evaluate patients with a generalized assessment.

Two of the large-scale studies of hand burns and functional outcome were done by Sheridan and colleagues,[1,2] one on children and the other on adults. The first followed 659 adults with hand burns and found that the large majority of hands regained normal function (97% of superficial and 81% of deep dermal and full-thickness injuries). This rate translates to 3% of superficial hand burns and 19% of deep dermal and full-thickness injuries not obtaining "normal" hand function. Assessment of "normal" was the judgment of the therapist or surgeon and was not based on any quantitative hand assessment.[1] Among those with joint capsule, bone, and extensor mechanism injuries, only 9% had "normal" hand function at follow-up evaluation. Eighty-one percent had abnormal joint motion but were independent in activities of daily living (ADL), and 9% were unable to perform ADL independently.[1]

In a review of a children's cohort of 495 patients (698 hand burns), "normal" functional recovery was also seen in the large majority of subjects (97% of second-degree and 85% of third-degree burns).[2] Two percent of hands with partial thickness burns and 9% of patients with full-thickness

Department of Physical Medicine and Rehabilitation, University of Texas Southwestern Medical Center, 5323 Harry Hines Boulevard, Dallas, TX 75390-9055, USA
E-mail address: karen.kowalske@utsouthwestern.edu

Hand Clin 25 (2009) 557–561
doi:10.1016/j.hcl.2009.06.003

burns did not have normal function but could perform ADL. Two percent of hands with partial thickness burns and 6% with full-thickness burns could not perform ADL.[2] This challenges the generalization that "all" partial- and full-thickness hand burns do well. Clinicians need to be reminded that although most patients with partial- or full-thickness hand burns recover well, there is still a percentage of patients who have significant impairment after this depth of burn.

In this same pediatric population, of those with associated bone and tendon injury only 20% attained "normal" hand function. A total of 51% did not have normal hand function but were able to perform ADL with equipment and 25% were not independent in ADL. If an amputation was performed, no hands were "normal." Half were independent in ADL with equipment and half were not. No formal assessment of range of motion or function was performed.[2]

In a smaller study, Nuchtern and colleagues[3] evaluated 25 patients (35 hands) with full-thickness hand burns. Eleven had Kirschner wire immobilization and grafting; there were 33 amputations performed in 21 of the hands, including 1 above the elbow, 5 below the elbow, and 15 at the level of the metacarpal phalangeal joint (MP). Outcome evaluation demonstrated severe impairment in 7 hands, 7 with moderate impairment, and 11 with minor sequelae. Again, no quantifiable tests were performed.[3]

RANGE OF MOTION AND STRENGTH

The hands represent the most common location of loss of range of motion in patients with burns. Several studies have shown a direct relationship between burn wound size and number of digit contractures.[4] This outcome makes intuitive sense as those with bigger burns are likely to have deeper hand burns, and these hand burns are less likely to be grafted within the first week.[4] The percentage of patients with contracture after hand burn varies from 16% to 23%[5,6] of patients admitted to hospital with a major burn injury. The most common contractures include wrist extension and flexion, index finger proximal interphalangeal joint (PIP) flexion, and MP flexion. According to the study by Schneider and colleagues,[6] most contractures are mild (48%) or moderate (42%) in severity with a relatively even distribution of involvement of each of the five digits (12%–17%). Other studies show contractures in 44% of those with third-degree burns and 6% of those with second-degree burns.[7] Understanding the rate of contracture does shed some light on how individuals recover after

hand burn, but does not shed light on the issue of function after hand burn.

The largest challenge with assessing individual joint range of motion is that the volume of data (30+ measurements per hand) creates a significant problem in analysis and interpretation. This issue is not easily overcome. To help with dealing with this volume of data, several investigators have used total active motion (TAM).[8–11] This technique adds the flexion and extension range with a loss of full range used as a negative number, giving a normal TAM of 260° for each finger. Johnson and colleagues describe using this tool for burn patients and suggest the following classification system: poor (<180°), good (180–219°), excellent (220–259°), and normal (260°). Unfortunately these investigators do not carry out any actual patient assessments, questionnaires, or measurements. Johnson and colleagues[8] also report that most outcome tools used have not been validated for burn injury, and that it is unclear whether they are sensitive to the issues burn patients have and whether they are responsive to progress in hand function over time.

One series that used TAM to evaluate 83 hand burns found an average total active motion of 230° 3 months after injury.[9] Another study found a mean TAM of 225° with normal pinch but decreased grip strength for patients with deep partial- or full-thickness hand burns that were grafted.[10]

Studies of fourth-degree hand burns show significant impairment of TAM with 40% or more having TAM scores less than 180°.[11] This is clearly a significant functional loss. Within this group, surgical reconstruction can have a significant impact, with surgery on those with virtually no range of motion having a "satisfactory" recovery after surgery.[12] Dorsal reconstruction can also improve TAM up to 120° in this group.[12] Reconstruction using a dorsal ulnar cutaneous flap can increase joint extension of about 75° for the MP and 105° for the PIP with subsequent significant improvement in grasp.[13] Abdominal flaps have also been used for reconstruction of the severely burned hand. This procedure can increase joint extension up to 75° for the MP and 105° for the PIP. Surprisingly, flap bulk does not seem to interfere with grasping (see Yongwei and colleagues[14]).

Although using TAM simplifies the statistics for study individuals with complex loss of range of motion of the hand, this method certainly falls short in truly describing the outcomes. The main challenge of this method is that lacking 20° of extension at the MP is not equivalent to having only 70° of flexion at the MP yet in the TAM methodology these two are evaluated as equivalent.

The only way to overcome this barrier may be by using computer-aided motion analysis of functional tasks with markers on each joint. This method may be able to provide the data needed to say that, for instance, an individual must have a specific amount of MP flexion of digits two and three for the act of grabbing a soda can, or a specific amount of MP and PIP extension is required for receiving change back from a cashier. One would also be able to tell if an amputation of the third digit limits function more than a severe boutonnière deformity. Unfortunately, these studies have not yet been done but would certainly help us better understand the role of scar contracture, capsular tightness, tendon rupture, and amputation in the overall level of function after burn injury to the hand.

Another technique for describing the hand is more descriptive and is based on the type of deformity. A list described by Salsbury includes first webspace adduction contracture, webspace contractures, dorsal skin contractures, fifth finger abduction deformity, MP joint extension deformities, extensor tendon adhesions, boutonnière deformity, PIP flexion deformities, median and ulnar nerve compression syndrome, amputation secondary to ischemic gangrene, elbow and axillary contractures, and heterotopic ossification of the elbow or wrist.[15] This list is certainly clinically useful but the impact on function is not clear. In clinical terms, hands with multiple boutonnière deformities are more functional than hands with PIP extension contractures. This fact is difficult for patients to understand. Many patients request surgical reconstruction for a more normal appearing hand with straight fingers. The burn care provider needs to help patients understand how this position may significantly limit functional grip.

Deep full-thickness hand burns can be catastrophic. One study of patients with this burn depth found 46% digit amputation, with 31% requiring amputation of more than one digit. Joint ankylosis was seen in 25% and 22% had a boutonnière deformity. A swan-neck deformity was seen in 9%, and 9% had joint subluxation. Mallet finger deformity was seen in 3% of this sample. Grip strength was 55% of normal for men and 61% of normal for women. Pinch strength was 55% of normal for men and 42% of normal for women.[11] These results demonstrate that this depth of burn clearly produces an impairment of much greater severity than hand burns that do not involve tendon, muscle, or bone.

SPECIFIC TESTS

There are many tests for evaluating hand function, very few of which have been validated in burn patients or used to evaluate function after hand burn. The Jebsen Hand Test, which includes writing, turning over a 3×5 card, picking up small objects, simulated feeding, stacking checkers, picking up large light objects, and picking up large heavy objects, is one of the few tests that has been used to study burn outcome.[16] This test was used to assess long-term functional evaluation of 88 patients with hand burns of uncertain depth.[17] Eighty percent of hands had normal function on all seven tasks. Sixteen percent of the hands demonstrated impaired function by showing a slower than predicted response of one or more component. Amputation, age, hand surface area, and total body surface area (TBSA) with third-degree burns were the significant predictors of hand function. There were no correlations with the timing of grafting. Patients were not sorted based on exposed tendon or bone.[17]

The Michigan Hand Questionnaire (MHQ) and Test d'Evaluation des Membres Supérieurs des Personnes Agées (TEMPA) have been used to assess patients at hospital discharge.[18] The MHQ is a hand-specific patient questionnaire comprising 37 questions that are categorized into six scales including overall hand function, ADL, pain, work performance, aesthetics, and patient satisfaction with hand function. The TEMPA assesses grip strength, endurance, and simulated ADL. The MHQ revealed that 68% of patients reported impairments in hand function. Of these, 76% reported impairment of ADL and 59% impairment with work. Patient satisfaction with hand function correlated with work performance, aesthetics, pain, and ADL. The MHQ indicated more hand function limitation than the TEMPA. There was a significant correlation between the MHQ and TEMPA total scores.[18] Because burn depth for the test subjects was not given, these data are difficult to put into context when discussing outcomes with a particular patient. It is clear that most patients are satisfied with their outcome but most have some functional limitations at hospital discharge. Further investigation over time with subclassification by burn depth would provide the additional data needed to help the understanding of these outcomes.

Using the Jebsen Hand Test to study individuals with deep full-thickness hand burns showed scores worse than the norms, with the most significant difficulty seen in writing a sentence. Women do better with writing, turning cards, and picking up small objects. Men do better than women on lifting a heavy can. It was observed that women used their fingernails which helped with manipulating small objects, and men had larger hand span allowing them to lift the heavy can.[11] In the

MHQ, subjects with fourth-degree hand burns report the most difficulty in ADL such as turning a door knob, picking up a coin, turning a key in a lock, or holding a frying pan. Patients' perception of hand function correlates with what they are able to do functionally. Despite these challenges and impairments, almost half of the patients with fourth-degree hand burns are fully independent in ADL and able to work.[11]

The American Medical Association (AMA) has issued guidelines for the assessment of impairment. These guidelines are used to evaluate limitations in strength and range of motion as well as skin changes. One study of the guidelines showed impairment after major burn injury to be 17% to 20%.[19] Although hand impairment was not selected individually, almost half of the impairment was due to impairment of upper extremity function. In using the AMA guidelines for permanent impairment the hands represent 60% of the upper extremity, so it is likely that a significant portion of this impairment was due to limitations in hand function.[19]

COMMUNITY INTEGRATION AND RETURN TO WORK

Community integration and return to work are important outcome issues to burn survivors. Several studies have shown that burn survivors have significant problems in the area of home integration, social integration, and productivity.[20] Although burn severity (TBSA) is correlated with the productivity, it is surprisingly not correlated with home or social integration.[20] The specific effect of a hand burn was not assessed in this study but it is known that most patients with major burn injuries have involvement of the hands, so it can be inferred that hand burns may interfere with integration and productivity.

Return to work is clearly an important milestone for patients with burn injuries. One study of 316 patients reported a mean return to work of 2 months. Surprisingly, in this study having a hand burn did not determine the timing of return to work.[21] Another study of 303 individuals who were working at the time of their burn injury found that 66% were working at a 6-month follow-up, and 90% were employed at 2 years following injury. The mean time off from work was 17 weeks. In this study, hand burn was a predictor of return to work along with psychiatry history and size of burn.[22] Specifically, those with an arm burn were 73% less likely to return to work at 6 months. In evaluating return to work rates in patients with hand burns (mean TBSA 14%), Umraw and colleagues[18] found that 90% of the patients returned to the same job after the injury (17% of these patients had some modification to their job description) at a mean of 18 months post injury. The main limitation of this study was the low patient number (N = 20).

In looking at barriers to return to work, it is clear that physical functioning has an impact on return to work throughout the course of recovery. This functionality includes the effect of having a hand burn.[23] Therefore, specific programs emphasizing physical functioning soon after burn injury may help facilitate return to work.

SUMMARY

From this review, it is clear that most patients with partial- and full-thickness hand burns do well but a small number do have limitations that need to be specifically addressed. It is also true that patients with involvement of tendon and bone have significantly more impairment but despite this impairment, many of these patients are reasonably functional, to the extent of being independent in ADL and able to return to work.

There are several important logistical considerations that need to be addressed to effectively study many of the issues discussed here. The development of rigorous studies that will provide meaningful results is contingent on clearly defining the patient population of study, and having well-defined outcome parameters and tools that can effectively capture them. There is an overwhelming volume of impairment data that can be collected including individual joint active and passive motion, hand strength, nerve conduction studies, and sensation thresholds, but as yet the correlation between results of these tests and hand function has not been defined. In addition, issues of disability (what activities an individual cannot accomplish) are also important. Lastly, it is critically important that the clinician asks burn survivors for their input regarding appearance, function, and quality of life. These data will help the health care community have a better understanding of the approach to dealing with the burned hand initially (ie, is it better to amputate or have a fused digit) and to facilitate the best possible outcomes for the patients.

REFERENCES

1. Sheridan RL, Hurley J, Smith MA, et al. The acutely burned hand: management and outcome based on a ten-year experience with 1047 acute hand burns. J Trauma 1995;38:406–11.
2. Sheridan RL, Baryza MJ, Pessina MA, et al. Acute hand burns in children: management and long-term

outcomes based on a 10 year experience with 698 injured hands. Ann Surg 1999;229(40):558–63.

3. Nuchtern JG, Engrav LH, Nakamura DY, et al. Treatment of fourth-degree hand burns. J Burn Care Rehabil 1995;16(1):36–42.

4. Kraemer MD, Jones T, Deitch EA. Burn contractures: incidence, predisposing factors, and results of surgical therapy. J Burn Care Rehabil 1988;9(3):261–5.

5. Antonopulos D, Danikas D, Dotsikas R, et al. The treatment of early and late hand contractures following burn injury (1978–1991). Ann MBC 1992;30:100–1.

6. Schneider JC, Holavanahalli R, Helm P, et al. Contractures in burn injury part II: investigating joints of the hand. J Burn Care Rehabil 2008;29(4):606–13.

7. Dobbs ER, Curreri W. Burns: analysis of physical therapy in 681 patients. J Trauma 1972;12:242–8.

8. Johnson C, Engrav LH, Heimbach DM, et al. Evaluating functional hand results after deep dermal burns with total active motion measurements. J Burn Care Rehabil 1980;1:19–21.

9. Barillo DJ, Harvey KD, Hobbs CL, et al. Prospective outcome analysis of a protocol for the surgical and rehabilitative management of burns to the hands. Plast Reconstr Surg 1997;100:1442–51.

10. Cartotto R. The burned hand: optimizing long-term outcomes with a standardized approach to acute and subacute care. Clin Plast Surg 2005;32:515–27.

11. Holavanahalli RK, Helm PA, Gorman AR, et al. Outcomes after deep full-thickness hand burns. Arch Phys Med Rehabil 2007;88(12 Suppl 2):S30–5.

12. Woo SH, Seul JH. Optimizing the correction of severe postburn hand deformities by using aggressive contracture releases and fasciocutaneous free-tissue transfers. Plast Reconstr Surg 2001;107(1):1–8.

13. Ulkar E, Uygur F, Karagoz H, et al. Flap choices to treat complex severe postburn hand contracture. Ann Plast Surg 2007;58(5):479–83.

14. Yongwei P, Jianing W, Junhui Z, et al. The abdominal flap using scarred skin in treatment of postburn hand deformities of severe burn patients. J Hand Surg Am 2004;29(2):2009–15.

15. Salisbury RE. Reconstruction of the burned hand. Clin Plast Surg 2000;27:65–9.

16. Jebsen RH. A objective standardized test of hand function. Arch Phys Med Rehabil 1969;50:311–9.

17. van Zuijlen PP, Kreis RW, Vloemans AF, et al. The prognostic factors regarding long-term functional outcome of full-thickness hand burns. Burns 1999;25:709–14.

18. Umraw N, Chan Y, Gomez M, et al. Effective hand function assessment after burn injuries. J Burn Care Rehabil 2004;25:134–9 [discussion: 128].

19. Costa BA, Engrav LH, Holavanahalli R, et al. Impairment after burns: a two-center, prospective report. Burns 2003;29:671–5.

20. Esselman PC, Ptacek JT, Kowalske KJ, et al. Community integration after burn injuries. J Burn Care Rehabil 2001;22(3):221–7.

21. Tanttula K, Vuola J, Asko-Seljavaara S. Return to employment after burn. Burns 1997;23:341–4.

22. Brych SB, Engrav LH, Rivara FP, et al. Time off work and return to work rates after burns: systematic review of the literature and a large two-center series. J Burn Care Rehabil 2001;22(6):401–5.

23. Esselman PC, Askay SW, Carroughter GJ, et al. Barriers to return to work after burn injury. Arch Phys Med Rehabil 2007;88(12):S50–6.

Index

doi:10.1016/S0749-0712(09)00085-7

hand.theclinics.com

United States Postal Service

Statement of Ownership, Management, and Circulation
(All Periodicals Publications Except Requestor Publications)

1. Publication Title	2. Publication Number	3. Filing Date
Hand Clinics	0 0 0 - 7 0 9	9/15/09

4. Issue Frequency	5. Number of Issues Published Annually	6. Annual Subscription Price
Feb, May, Aug, Nov	4	$282.00

7. Complete Mailing Address of Known Office of Publication (Not printer) (Street, city, county, state, and ZIP+4®)

Elsevier Inc.
360 Park Avenue South
New York, NY 10010-1710

Contact Person
Stephen Busting
Telephone: (Include area code)
215-239-3688

8. Complete Mailing Address of Headquarters or General Business Office of Publisher (Not printer)

Elsevier Inc., 360 Park Avenue South, New York, NY 10010-1710

9. Full Names and Complete Mailing Addresses of Publisher, Editor, and Managing Editor (Do not leave blank)
Publisher (Name and complete mailing address)

John Schrefer, Elsevier, Inc., 1600 John F. Kennedy Blvd. Suite 1800, Philadelphia, PA 19103-2899

Editor (Name and complete mailing address)

Deb Dellapena, Elsevier, Inc., 1600 John F. Kennedy Blvd. Suite 1800, Philadelphia, PA 19103-2899

Managing Editor (Name and complete mailing address)

Catherine Bewick, Elsevier, Inc., 1600 John F. Kennedy Blvd. Suite 1800, Philadelphia, PA 19103-2899

10. Owner (Do not leave blank. If the publication is owned by a corporation, give the name and address of the corporation immediately followed by the names and addresses of all stockholders owning or holding 1 percent or more of the total amount of stock. If not owned by a corporation, give the names and addresses of the individual owners. If owned by a partnership or other unincorporated firm, give its name and address as well as those of each individual owner. If the publication is published by a nonprofit organization, give its name and address.)

Full Name	Complete Mailing Address
Wholly owned subsidiary of	4520 East-West Highway
Reed/Elsevier, US holdings	Bethesda, MD 20814

11. Known Bondholders, Mortgagees, and Other Security Holders Owning or Holding 1 Percent or More of Total Amount of Bonds, Mortgages, or Other Securities. If none, check box ☐ None

Full Name	Complete Mailing Address
N/A	

12. Tax Status (For completion by nonprofit organizations authorized to mail at nonprofit rates) (Check one)
The purpose, function, and nonprofit status of this organization and the exempt status for federal income tax purposes:
☐ Has Not Changed During Preceding 12 Months
☐ Has Changed During Preceding 12 Months (Publisher must submit explanation of change with this statement)

PS Form 3526, September 2007 (Page 1 of 3 (Instructions Page 3)) PSN 7530-01-000-9931 PRIVACY NOTICE: See our Privacy policy in www.usps.com

---

13. Publication Title	14. Issue Date for Circulation Data Below
Hand Clinics	August 2009

15. Extent and Nature of Circulation		Average No. Copies Each Issue During Preceding 12 Months	No. Copies of Single Issue Published Nearest to Filing Date
a. Total Number of Copies (Net press run)		2123	2000
b. Paid Circulation (By Mail and Outside the Mail)	(1) Mailed Outside-County Paid Subscriptions Stated on PS Form 3541. (Include paid distribution above nominal rate, advertiser's proof copies, and exchange copies)	1141	1107
	(2) Mailed In-County Paid Subscriptions Stated on PS Form 3541 (Include paid distribution above nominal rate, advertiser's proof copies, and exchange copies)		
	(3) Paid Distribution Outside the Mails Including Sales Through Dealers and Carriers, Street Vendors, Counter Sales, and Other Paid Distribution Outside USPS®	419	406
	(4) Paid Distribution by Other Classes Mailed Through the USPS (e.g. First-Class Mail®)		
c. Total Paid Distribution (Sum of 15b (1), (2), (3), and (4)) ▶		1560	1513
d. Free or Nominal Rate Distribution (By Mail and Outside the Mail)	(1) Free or Nominal Rate Outside-County Copies Included on PS Form 3541	80	68
	(2) Free or Nominal Rate In-County Copies Included on PS Form 3541		
	(3) Free or Nominal Rate Copies Mailed at Other Classes Through the USPS (e.g. First-Class Mail)		
	(4) Free or Nominal Rate Distribution Outside the Mail (Carriers or other means)		
e. Total Free or Nominal Rate Distribution (Sum of 15d (1), (2), (3) and (4)) ▶		80	68
f. Total Distribution (Sum of 15c and 15e) ▶		1640	1581
g. Copies not Distributed (See instructions to publishers #4 (page #3)) ▶		483	419
h. Total (Sum of 15f and g) ▶		2123	2000
i. Percent Paid (15c divided by 15f times 100)		95.12%	95.70%

16. Publication of Statement of Ownership
☐ If the publication is a general publication, publication of this statement is required. Will be printed in the November 2009 issue of this publication. ☐ Publication not required

17. Signature and Title of Editor, Publisher, Business Manager, or Owner	Date
Stephen R. Bushing Stephen R. Bushing – Subscription Services Coordinator	September 15, 2009

I certify that all information furnished on this form is true and complete. I understand that anyone who furnishes false or misleading information on this form or who omits material or information requested on the form may be subject to criminal sanctions (including fines and imprisonment) and/or civil sanctions (including civil penalties).

PS Form 3526, September 2007 (Page 2 of 3)

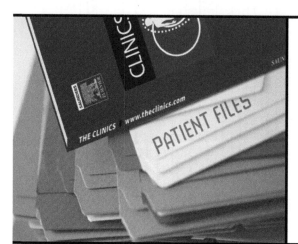
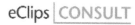
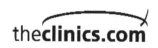

Moving?

Make sure your subscription moves with you!

To notify us of your new address, find your **Clinics Account Number** (located on your mailing label above your name), and contact customer service at:

Email: journalscustomerservice-usa@elsevier.com

800-654-2452 (subscribers in the U.S. & Canada)
314-447-8871 (subscribers outside of the U.S. & Canada)

Fax number: 314-447-8029

Elsevier Health Sciences Division
Subscription Customer Service
3251 Riverport Lane
Maryland Heights, MO 63043

*To ensure uninterrupted delivery of your subscription, please notify us at least 4 weeks in advance of move.

ELSEVIER

Printed and bound by CPI Group (UK) Ltd, Croydon, CR0 4YY

03/10/2024

01040353-0013